ANTI-CANCER DIET COOKBOOK

Transform Your Kitchen With Comforting And Nourishing Recipes To Boost Your Immune System And Fight Cancer Naturally

LINDA DONLEY

TABLE OF CONTENTS

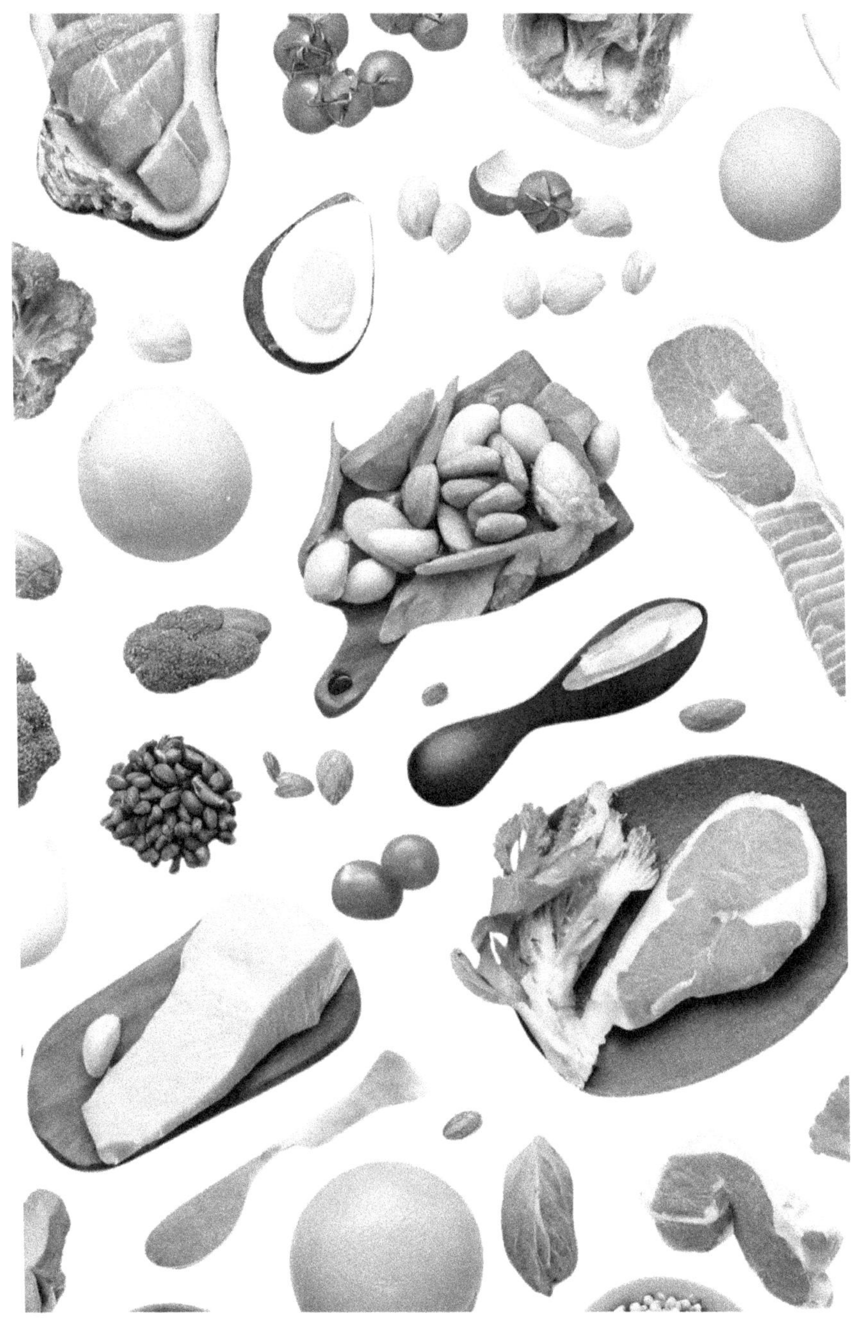

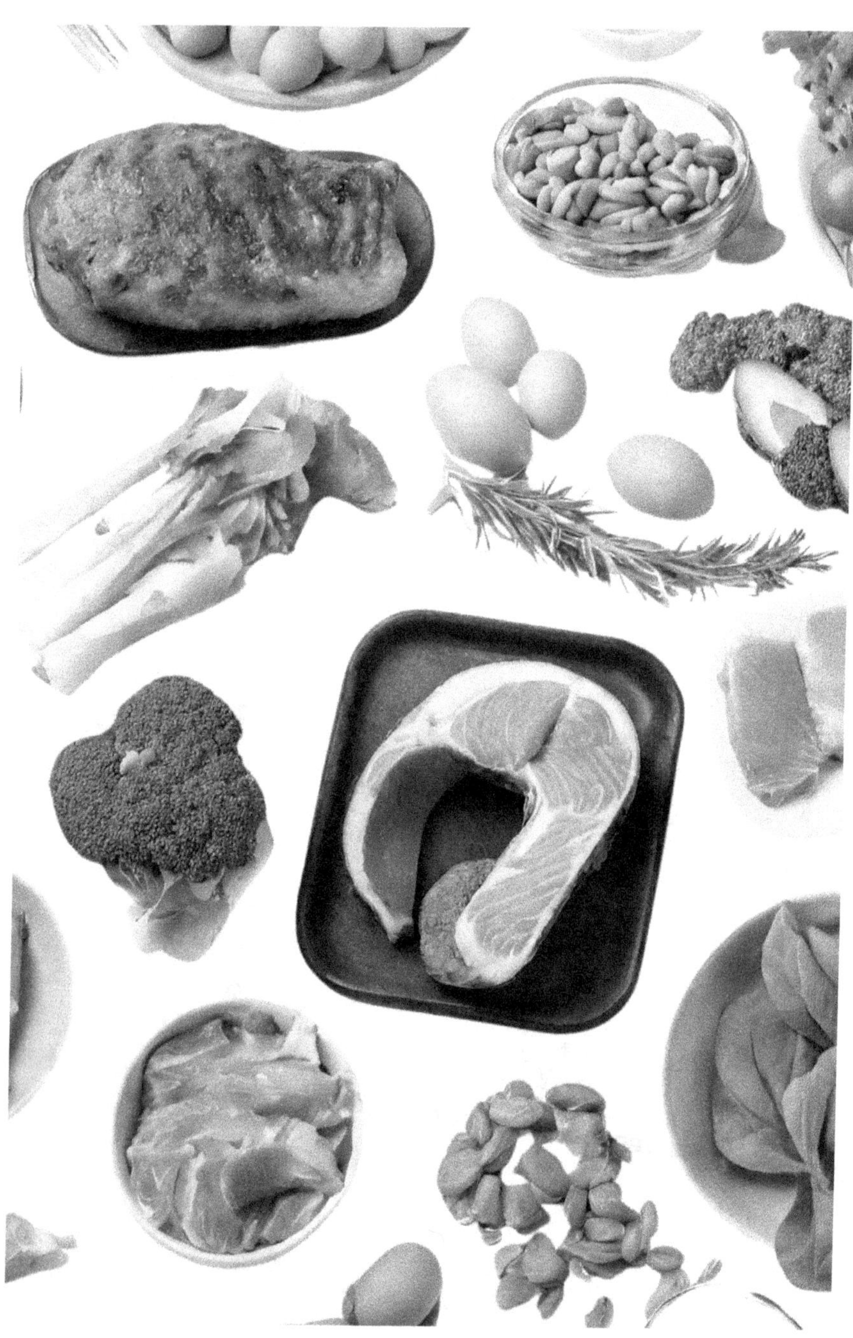

As I write this book, I am reminded of an experience that forever impacted my life. It's a tale of perseverance, optimism, and the wonderful power of food to overcome hardship.

It all started when my dear sister, Rebecca, got a dreadful cancer diagnosis. The news shook our world, sending us into a state of terror and uncertainty. But, despite the gloom, there remained a ray of hope: the steadfast will to battle, conquer, and prosper.

I recall spending numerous hours at Rebecca's side, understanding the complexity of her treatment plan and providing whatever assistance I could. We went on a voyage of exploration, looking into every option to supplement her medical treatment and boost her strength.

In the middle of the pandemonium, one bright spot emerged: food's transforming ability. Through painstaking investigation and testing, we discovered a plethora of information concerning the function of diet in cancer prevention and treatment. Armed with this newfound knowledge, we set out to maximize the healing potential of each component and meal.

Rebecca's path, full of trials and triumphs, became a testimonial to the significant influence of an anti-cancer diet. Her body felt energized and alive after each healthy meal. As her strength rose, so did our trust in food's transformational ability as medicine.

The concept for this book sprang from a profoundly personal event. I wanted to share our story, including the hardships, successes, and essential lessons learned along the road. More than anything, I wanted to provide hope and assistance to people going on their cancer journey.

The following sections include a treasure mine of recipes, thoughts, and practical advice to help you on your recovery journey. Whether you're dealing with a cancer diagnosis yourself or supporting a loved one, this book provides a road map to greater health, one delicious meal at a time.

Unlocking the Healing Potential of Nutrition: Welcome to Your Anti-Cancer Kitchen

Medical advances have had a substantial impact on the fight against cancer. However, despite the abundance of therapies available, one potent instrument that is sometimes forgotten is the kitchen. "Welcome to Your Anti-Cancer Kitchen" is more than just another cookbook; it's a thorough guide that reveals how dietary choices may have a significant influence on cancer prevention and treatment. This article explores how this cookbook uses the power of nutrition to empower people in their battle against cancer.

Research has repeatedly shown that nutrition plays a crucial role in avoiding cancer. Welcome to Your Anti-Cancer Kitchen explores this link by giving evidence-based insights into how individual foods and dietary habits might affect cancer development and progression. The cookbook teaches readers how to include cancer-fighting elements into their regular meals, including antioxidant-rich fruits and vegetables, anti-inflammatory spices, and herbs. Furthermore, it highlights the necessity of eating a well-balanced diet to strengthen the immune system and promote general health, both of which are critical elements in cancer prevention.

How Can This Cookbook Help You Fight Cancer?

Nutrient-rich foods: Welcome to Your Anti-Cancer Kitchen is full of tasty, nutrient-dense foods that will feed both your body and spirit. Each dish is carefully designed to contain components renowned for their cancer-fighting characteristics, such as cruciferous veggies, berries, and healthy grains. From vivid salads to substantial soups and tasty main meals, the cookbook shows that healthy eating can be both pleasurable and gratifying.

Empowering Education: In addition to recipes, the cookbook provides a complete resource for learning the science behind cancer prevention via diet. It teaches readers about the advantages of various nutrients and phytochemicals, allowing them to make more educated dietary decisions. The cookbook empowers people to take charge of their health and well-being by explaining complicated dietary principles in simple terms.

Practical Tips & Strategies: Recognizing that adopting a cancer-fighting diet might be difficult, Welcome to Your Anti-Cancer Kitchen offers practical advice and methods to help you move to a healthier lifestyle. Whether it's meal planning assistance, grocery shopping recommendations, or easy culinary methods, the cookbook provides readers with the resources they need to confidently and easily manage their anti-cancer path.

This cookbook promotes a comprehensive approach to cancer prevention and treatment. It urges readers to include other lifestyle variables in their health regimen, such as regular physical exercise, stress management, and appropriate sleep. By addressing the complex aspect of health, the cookbook encourages holistic techniques for cancer prevention and general well-being.

Welcome to Your Anti-Cancer. Kitchen goes beyond the traditional limitations of a cookbook, emerging as a source of hope and empowerment for cancer patients. The cookbook provides a path to greater health and resilience in the face of tragedy by emphasizing the healing power of food and combining practical advice with holistic ideas. By accepting the teachings contained inside its pages, readers may start on a transforming journey to a better, cancer-free future.

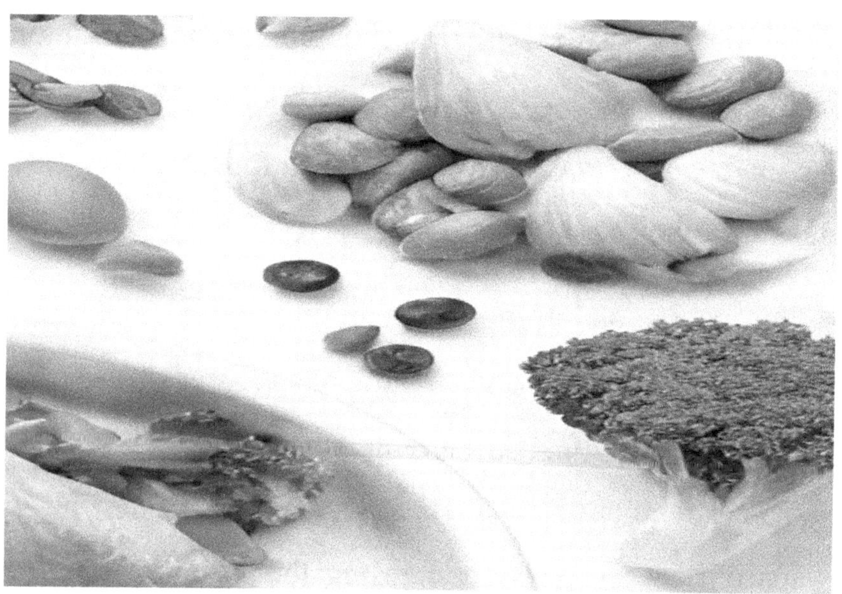

CHAPTER ONE

What Is the Anti-Cancer Diet?

An anti-cancer diet is a nutritional strategy that aims to lower the risk of cancer formation, aid in cancer therapy, and improve general well-being. It stresses eating complete, nutrient-dense foods while limiting or eliminating processed and possibly hazardous ingredients. The basic idea behind an anti-cancer diet is to use food's inherent therapeutic capabilities to foster a healthy internal environment and counteract variables that lead to cancer development and progression.

Key Principles of Anticancer Nutrition

Plant-based foods, such as fruits and vegetables, whole grains, legumes, nuts, and seeds, are essential for an anti-cancer diet. These foods are high in vitamins, minerals, antioxidants, and phytochemicals, which have powerful anti-inflammatory and cancer-fighting qualities. Fill your plate with a wide variety of plant foods to optimize their health benefits and promote healthy cellular function.

Prioritize Plant chemicals, often known as phytonutrients, may be found in fruits, vegetables, herbs, and spices. These chemicals have an important role in cell protection, tumor development inhibition, and immune function modulation. Include a variety of phytonutrient-rich foods in your diet, such as cruciferous vegctables (e.g., broccoli, kale), berries, turmeric, garlic, and green tea, to maximize their cancer-fighting potential.

Choose Healthy Fats: Avocados, olive oil, nuts, seeds, and fatty seafood like salmon provide critical nutrients that support numerous biological activities. Omega-3 fatty acids, in particular, have anti-inflammatory characteristics and may lower the risk of some malignancies. Limit your intake of saturated and trans fats found in processed and fried meals, since they may cause inflammation and contribute to cancer development.

Limiting processed and red meat consumption has been associated with an increased risk of cancer, especially colon cancer. Examples include bacon, sausage, and deli meats. Reduce your intake of these items and instead go for lean protein sources such as chicken, fish, tofu, lentils, and plant-based alternatives. When it comes to meat, aim for high-quality organic selections and consume in moderation.

Consuming too much added sugars and refined carbs, such as those found in sugary drinks, candies, pastries, and grains, may lead to inflammation, insulin resistance, and weight gain, all of which are risk factors for cancer. Instead, choose full, unprocessed carbs such as fruits, vegetables, whole grains, and legumes, which give fiber, vitamins, minerals, and long-lasting energy without the bad health consequences of refined carbohydrates.

Stock Your Pantry for Success: Consume a varied range of fresh fruits and vegetables in a rainbow of hues for optimal nutrition. Stock your refrigerator with leafy greens, cruciferous veggies, berries, citrus fruits, and other seasonal items to use in meals and snacks.

Choose whole grains like brown rice, quinoa, oats, barley, and whole wheat pasta to get fiber, vitamins, minerals, and sustained energy. To improve general health and lower the risk of cancer, replace processed grains with whole grains.

Include legumes like beans, lentils, and chickpeas in your cupboard to boost plant-based protein, fiber, and phytonutrients in your meals. These adaptable components may be used in soups, stews, salads, and side dishes to boost nutrition and satiety.

Choose healthy fats like olive oil, avocado oil, nuts, seeds, and fatty seafood to promote heart health and minimize inflammation. Use these fats in cooking, salad dressings, and snacking to improve general health.

Stock up on herbs, spices, and seasonings to add flavor and nutrition to your food.

Turmeric, ginger, garlic, cinnamon, and cayenne pepper are just a handful of the powerful anti-inflammatory and antioxidant-rich components that may improve your meals.

An anti-cancer diet includes the basic premise of utilizing food as medicine to improve health, prevent illness, and aid in healing. By adopting a plant-based, nutrient-dense diet and implementing fundamental anti-cancer nutrition concepts into your everyday life, you can empower yourself to take proactive actions toward lowering your risk of cancer and improving your overall well-being. Stocking your cupboard with good, nourishing products sets the stage for a lifetime of health and vigor.

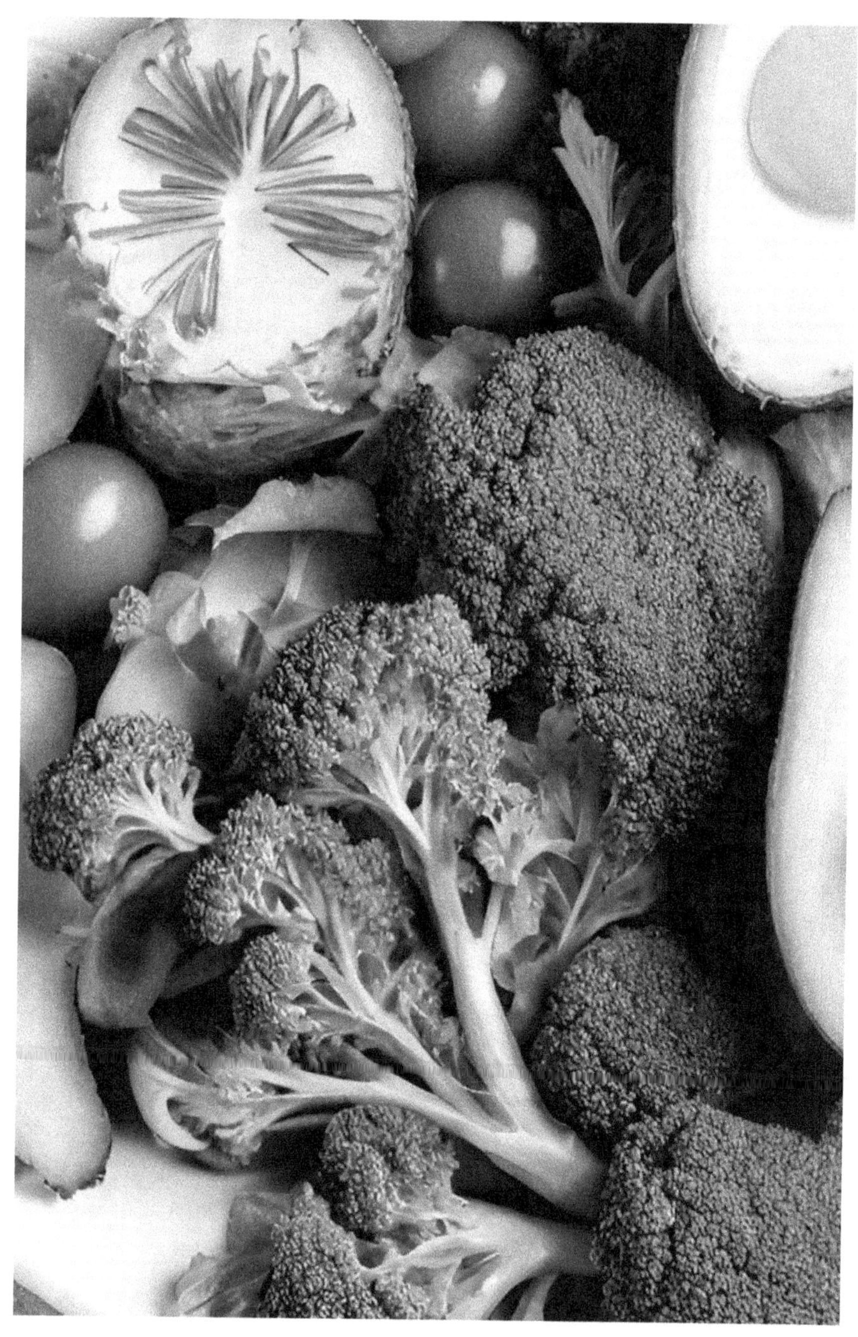

CHAPTER TWO

Superfoods for Cancer Prevention

Cancer prevention is a complicated task that requires a comprehensive approach to health and well-being. While genetics and environmental variables contribute to cancer development, a new study indicates that dietary choices might have a significant influence on cancer risk. Incorporating nutrient-dense superfoods into your diet is an effective way to strengthen your body's natural defenses and lower your risk of cancer. This article looks at some of nature's most powerful cancer-fighting superfoods and how to include them in a healthy, anti-cancer diet.

Explore Nature's Cancer Fighters:

Superfoods are nutrient-dense foods that are especially helpful to health and well-being because they include a high concentration of vitamins, minerals, antioxidants, and phytochemicals. Many of these superfoods contain special qualities that have been demonstrated to slow cancer development, decrease inflammation, and improve general cellular health. By including these powerful substances in your diet, you may take advantage of nature's arsenal of cancer fighters to strengthen your body's defenses and improve overall health.

Include Berries and Other Antioxidant-Rich Foods:

Berries including blueberries, strawberries, raspberries, and blackberries are known for their high antioxidant content, making them powerful friends in the battle against cancer. Antioxidants aid in neutralizing damaging free radicals, which may damage cells and DNA, possibly leading to cancer growth. In addition to berries, antioxidant-rich foods including pomegranates, cherries, and oranges may help protect against cancer. Incorporate these vivid fruits into your diet by eating them fresh as snacks, adding them to smoothies, or combining them into salads and desserts for a tasty and nutritional boost.

Harnessing the Power of Cruciferous Vegetables:

Cruciferous vegetables, such as broccoli, cauliflower, kale, Brussels sprouts, and cabbage, are known for their powerful anti-cancer qualities. These veggies include sulfur-containing chemicals known as glucosinolates, which have been demonstrated to suppress the development of cancer cells and promote detoxification in the body. Cruciferous vegetables are also high in vitamins, minerals, and fiber, making them an important part of a cancer-fighting diet. To gain the advantages of cruciferous vegetables, steam, roast, or sauté them as side dishes or mix them into soups, stir-fries, and salads.

Embracing Healthy Fats: Nuts, Seeds and Avocado

Healthy fats are important for maintaining general health and lowering the risk of cancer. Nuts, seeds, and avocados are high in healthful fats, including monounsaturated and polyunsaturated fats, as well as vital omega-3 fatty acids. These fats have been found to lower inflammation, promote heart health, and prevent cancer development and progression. Add a variety of nuts and seeds to your diet, such as almonds, walnuts, flaxseeds, and chia seeds, as snacks, salad and yogurt toppings, or components in homemade granola and energy bars. Avocado may also be used to add creaminess and nutrients to salads, sandwiches, and smoothies.

Whole grains play an important role in an anti-cancer diet.

Whole grains are vital for an anti-cancer diet because they include important elements including fiber, vitamins, minerals, and phytochemicals. Fiber-rich whole grains including oats, brown rice, quinoa, barley, and whole wheat promote digestive health, manage blood sugar levels, and lower the risk of colorectal cancer. Whole grains also include antioxidants and other bioactive substances, which have been found to slow cancer development and boost general health. To integrate more whole grains into your diet, choose whole-grain bread, pasta, and cereals, replace refined grains with whole-grain alternatives, and experiment with ancient grains like farro, millet, and teff when cooking and baking.

Putting these superfoods into your diet effectively lowers your risk of cancer while also increasing general health and wellness. Berries, cruciferous vegetables, nuts, seeds, avocado, and whole grains are just a handful of nature's cancer-fighting superfoods that may help guard against this deadly illness. By embracing these nutrient-dense foods and integrating them into a well-balanced, anti-cancer diet, you can set yourself up for a healthy, cancer-free future. So, let your plate be your medication and your kitchen be your pharmacy as you use superfoods to help you achieve your health and wellness goals.

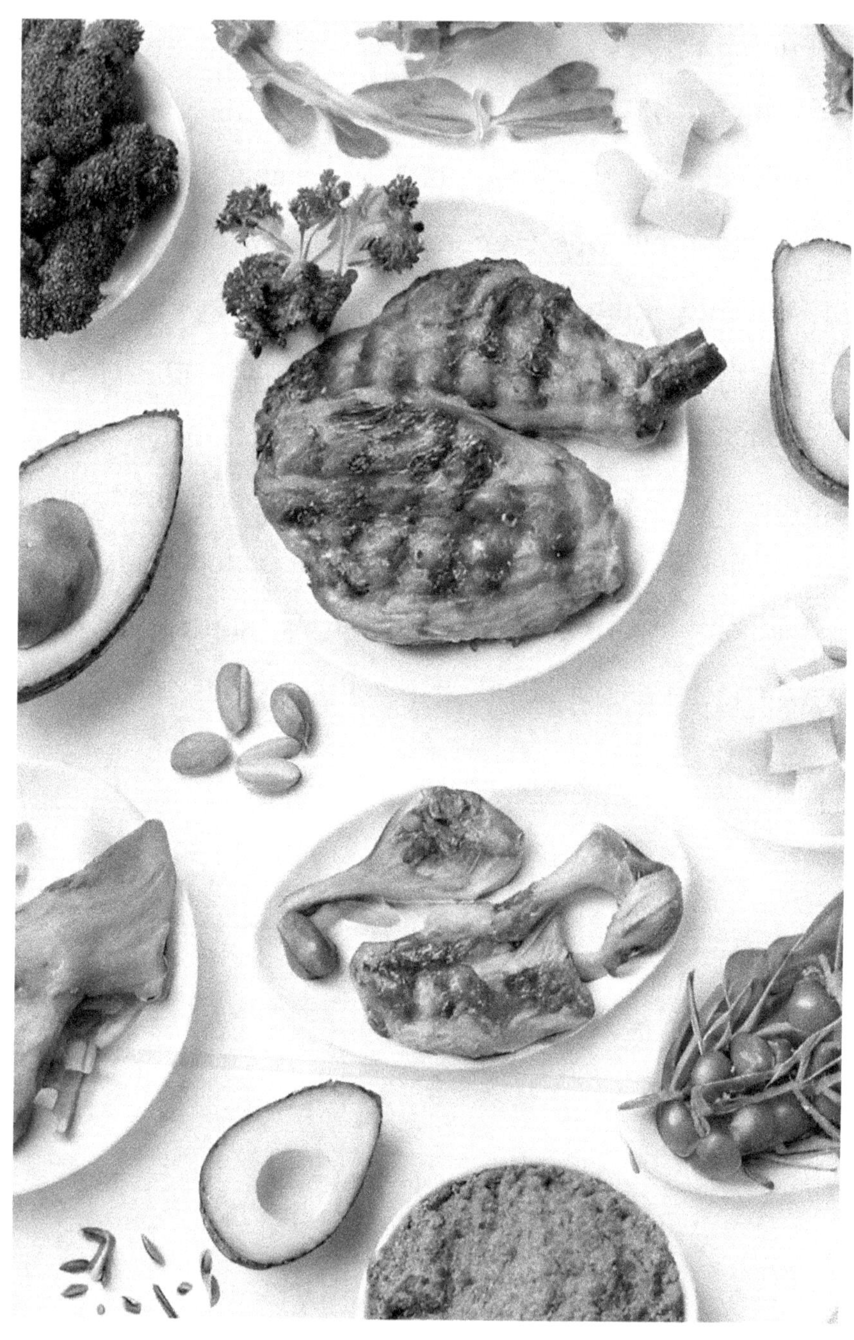

CHAPTER THREE

Breakfast Recipes

1. Berry Oatmeal Breakfast Bowl

- **Description:** A nutritious and antioxidant-rich breakfast bowl featuring vibrant berries and hearty oats to kickstart your day with a cancer-fighting boost.

- **Prep:** 5 minutes

- **Servings:** 1

- **Cooking Time:** 10 minutes

- **Nutritional Facts:** Approximately 300 calories per serving, high in fiber, vitamins, and antioxidants.

- **Ingredients:**

  - 1/2 cup rolled oats

  - 1 cup almond milk (or any preferred milk)

- 1/2 cup mixed berries (such as strawberries, blueberries, raspberries)

- 1 tablespoon chia seeds

- 1 tablespoon honey or maple syrup

- 1 tablespoon chopped nuts (almonds, walnuts, or pecans)

- **Instructions:**

1. In a saucepan, bring almond milk to a gentle boil.

2. Stir in rolled oats and reduce heat to low. Cook for about 5-7 minutes, stirring occasionally, until oats are tender and the mixture thickens.

3. Remove from heat and transfer oatmeal to a serving bowl.

4. Top with mixed berries, chia seeds, honey or maple syrup, and chopped nuts.

5. Enjoy warm.

2. Avocado Toast with Tomato and Basil

- **Description:** A simple yet satisfying breakfast option loaded with healthy fats from avocado and antioxidants from fresh tomatoes and basil.

- **Prep:** 5 minutes

- **Servings:** 1

- **Cooking Time:** 5 minutes

- **Nutritional Facts:** Approximately 250 calories per serving, rich in monounsaturated fats, vitamins, and minerals.

- **Ingredients:**

    - 1 ripe avocado

    - 2 slices whole grain bread

    - 1 small tomato, sliced

    - Fresh basil leaves

    - Salt and pepper to taste

- **Instructions:**

1.   Toast the whole grain bread slices until golden brown.

2.   Meanwhile, scoop out the flesh of the avocado and mash it with a fork in a small bowl. Season with salt and pepper to taste.

3.   Spread mashed avocado evenly onto the toasted bread slices.

4.   Top with sliced tomatoes and fresh basil leaves.

5.   Sprinkle with additional salt and pepper if desired.

6.   Serve immediately.

3. Green Smoothie Bowl

- **Description:** A refreshing and nutrient-packed breakfast bowl featuring leafy greens, tropical fruits, and superfood toppings for a vibrant start to your day.

- **Prep:** 5 minutes

- **Servings:** 1

- **Cooking Time:** 0 minutes

- **Nutritional Facts:** Approximately 200 calories per serving, high in fiber, vitamins, and antioxidants.

- **Ingredients:**

  - 1 cup spinach or kale

  - 1/2 frozen banana

  - 1/2 cup frozen pineapple chunks

  - 1/2 cup almond milk (or any preferred milk)

  - 1 tablespoon chia seeds

  - Toppings: sliced kiwi, shredded coconut, granola, sliced almonds

- **Instructions:**

1. In a blender, combine spinach or kale, frozen banana, frozen pineapple chunks, and almond milk.

2. Blend until smooth and creamy.

3. Pour the green smoothie into a bowl.

4. Top with sliced kiwi, shredded coconut, granola, and sliced almonds.

5. Serve immediately with a spoon.

4. Quinoa Breakfast Bowl with Mixed Berries

- **Description:** A protein-rich breakfast bowl featuring quinoa, mixed berries, and a touch of sweetness from maple syrup for a wholesome and satisfying morning meal.

- **Prep:** 10 minutes

- **Servings:** 2

- **Cooking Time:** 15 minutes

- **Nutritional Facts:** Approximately 350 calories per serving, high in protein, fiber, vitamins, and antioxidants.

- **Ingredients:**

  - 1/2 cup quinoa, rinsed

- 1 cup water

- 1/2 cup mixed berries (such as strawberries, blueberries, raspberries)

- 2 tablespoons chopped nuts (almonds, walnuts, or pecans)

- 2 tablespoons maple syrup

- **Instructions:**

1. In a saucepan, bring water to a boil. Add quinoa and reduce heat to low. Cover and simmer for about 12-15 minutes, or until quinoa is cooked and water is absorbed.

2. Fluff the cooked quinoa with a fork and divide it into serving bowls.

3. Top with mixed berries and chopped nuts.

4. Drizzle with maple syrup.

5. Serve warm and enjoy!

5. Greek Yogurt Parfait with Berries and Almonds

- **Description:** A protein-packed breakfast parfait featuring creamy Greek yogurt, antioxidant-rich berries, and crunchy almonds for a delicious and nutritious morning treat.

- **Prep:** 5 minutes

- **Servings:** 1

- **Cooking Time:** 0 minutes

- **Nutritional Facts:** Approximately 300 calories per serving, high in protein, vitamins, and antioxidants.

- **Ingredients:**

  - 1/2 cup plain Greek yogurt

  - 1/2 cup mixed berries (such as strawberries, blueberries, raspberries)

  - 1 tablespoon sliced almonds

  - 1 tablespoon honey or maple syrup

- **Instructions:**

1.   In a serving glass or bowl, layer Greek yogurt, mixed berries, and sliced almonds.

2.   Drizzle with honey or maple syrup.

3.   Repeat the layers until the glass or bowl is filled.

4.   Serve immediately as a delicious and nutritious breakfast or snack.

6. Whole Grain Pancakes with Banana and Walnuts

- **Description:** Fluffy whole grain pancakes topped with sliced banana, chopped walnuts, and a drizzle of honey for a hearty and satisfying breakfast that's packed with fiber and essential nutrients.

- **Prep:** 10 minutes

- **Servings:** 2

- **Cooking Time:** 15 minutes

- **Nutritional Facts:** Approximately 350 calories per serving, high in fiber, vitamins, and minerals.

- **Ingredients:**

  - 1 cup whole wheat flour

  - 1 tablespoon baking powder

  - 1/4 teaspoon salt

  - 1 tablespoon honey or maple syrup

  - 1 cup almond milk (or any preferred milk)

  - 1 egg

  - 1 ripe banana, sliced

  - 2 tablespoons chopped walnuts

- **Instructions:**

1. In a large mixing bowl, whisk together whole wheat flour, baking powder, and salt.

2. In a separate bowl, whisk together honey or maple syrup, almond milk, and egg.

3.   Pour the wet ingredients into the dry ingredients and stir until just combined. Do not overmix.

4.   Heat a non-stick skillet or griddle over medium heat. Lightly grease with cooking spray or a small amount of oil.

5.   Pour about 1/4 cup of batter onto the skillet for each pancake. Cook until bubbles form on the surface, then flip and cook until golden brown on the other side.

6.   Serve the pancakes warm, topped with sliced banana, chopped walnuts, and a drizzle of honey or maple syrup.

7. Spinach and Feta Egg Muffins

- **Description:** Protein-packed egg muffins loaded with nutritious spinach, tangy feta cheese, and flavorful herbs for a convenient and satisfying breakfast option.

- **Prep:** 10 minutes

- **Servings:** 6

- **Cooking Time:** 20 minutes

- **Nutritional Facts:** Approximately 150 calories per serving, high in protein, vitamins, and minerals.

- **Ingredients:**

  - 6 large eggs

  - 1 cup fresh spinach, chopped

  - 1/4 cup crumbled feta cheese

  - 2 tablespoons chopped fresh herbs (such as parsley, dill, or chives)

  - Salt and pepper to taste

- **Instructions:**

1. Preheat the oven to 350°F (175°C). Grease a muffin tin or line with paper liners.

2. In a large mixing bowl, whisk together eggs, chopped spinach, crumbled feta cheese, chopped herbs, salt, and pepper.

3.   Divide the egg mixture evenly among the muffin cups.

4.   Bake for 15-20 minutes, or until the egg muffins are set and lightly golden on top.

5.   Remove from the oven and let cool slightly before serving.

6.   Enjoy egg muffins warm or store them in the refrigerator for up to 3 days for a quick and convenient breakfast option.

8. Chia Seed Pudding with Mango and Coconut

- **Description:** Creamy chia seed pudding infused with tropical flavors from fresh mango and shredded coconut, perfect for a nutritious and satisfying breakfast or snack.

- **Prep:** 5 minutes (plus chilling time)

- **Servings:** 2

- **Cooking Time:** 0 minutes

- **Nutritional Facts:** Approximately 250 calories per serving, high in fiber, vitamins, and antioxidants.

- **Ingredients:**

    - 1/4 cup chia seeds

    - 1 cup coconut milk (or any preferred milk)

    - 1 ripe mango, diced

    - 2 tablespoons shredded coconut

    - Optional: honey or maple syrup for sweetness

- **Instructions:**

1.   In a mixing bowl, whisk together chia seeds and coconut milk. If desired, sweeten with honey or maple syrup to taste.

2.   Cover the bowl and refrigerate for at least 2 hours or overnight, until the chia pudding thickens and sets.

3.   To serve, divide the chia pudding into serving bowls or glasses.

4.   Top with diced mango and shredded coconut.

5.   Enjoy chilled as a refreshing and nutritious breakfast or snack.

9. Sweet Potato Breakfast Hash with Kale and Eggs

- **Description:** A hearty and flavorful breakfast hash featuring nutrient-rich sweet potatoes, leafy kale, and protein-packed eggs for a satisfying start to your day.

- **Prep:** 10 minutes

- **Servings:** 2

- **Cooking Time:** 20 minutes

- **Nutritional Facts:** Approximately 300 calories per serving, high in fiber, vitamins, and protein.

- **Ingredients:**

  - 1 large sweet potato, peeled and diced

  - 1 tablespoon olive oil

- 2 cups chopped kale

- 2 eggs

- Salt and pepper to taste

- **Instructions:**

1. Heat olive oil in a large skillet over medium heat. Add diced sweet potato and cook for 8-10 minutes, stirring occasionally, until tender and lightly browned.

2. Add chopped kale to the skillet and cook for an additional 3-5 minutes, until wilted.

3. Create two wells in the sweet potato and kale mixture. Crack an egg into each well.

4. Cover the skillet and cook for 5-7 minutes, or until the eggs are cooked to your desired doneness.

5. Season with salt and pepper to taste.

6. Serve the sweet potato breakfast hash hot, garnished with fresh herbs if desired.

10. Overnight Oats with Peanut Butter and Banana

- **Description:** Creamy and indulgent overnight oats infused with the flavors of peanut butter and banana for a delicious and convenient breakfast option that's perfect for busy mornings.

- **Prep:** 5 minutes (plus chilling time)

- **Servings:** 1

- **Cooking Time:** 0 minutes

- **Nutritional Facts:** Approximately 400 calories per serving, high in fiber, protein, and healthy fats.

- **Ingredients:**

    - 1/2 cup rolled oats

    - 1/2 cup almond milk (or any preferred milk)

    - 1 tablespoon peanut butter

    - 1/2 ripe banana, mashed

    - 1 tablespoon chia seeds

- Optional: honey or maple syrup for sweetness

- **Instructions:**

1. In a mason jar or airtight container, combine rolled oats, almond milk, peanut butter, mashed banana, and chia seeds. If desired, sweeten with honey or maple syrup to taste.

2. Stir well to combine all ingredients.

3. Cover the jar or container and refrigerate overnight or for at least 4 hours, until the oats have softened and absorbed the liquid.

4. To serve, give the overnight oats a good stir and top with additional banana slices, a drizzle of peanut butter, and a sprinkle of chia seeds.

5. Enjoy chilled as a convenient and nutritious breakfast option.

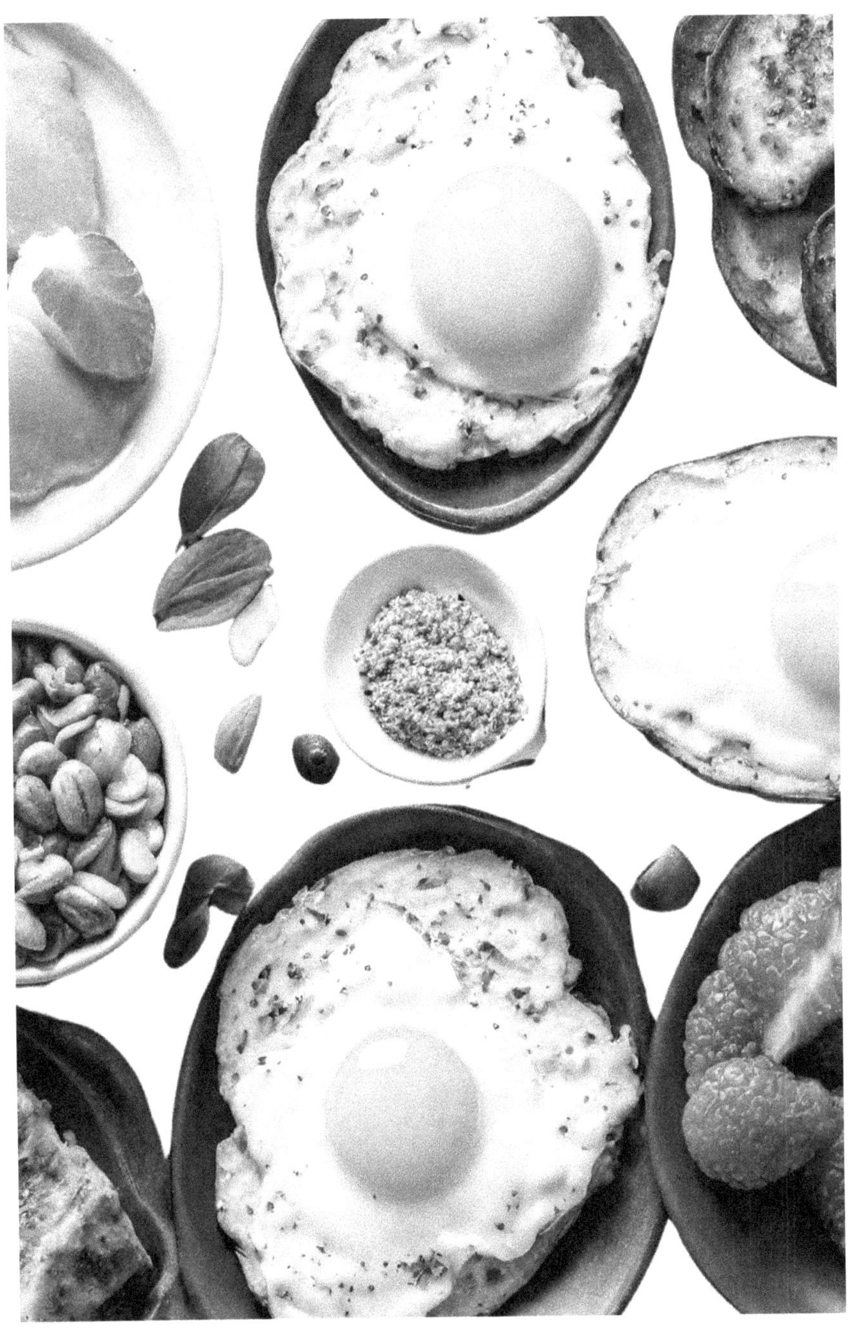

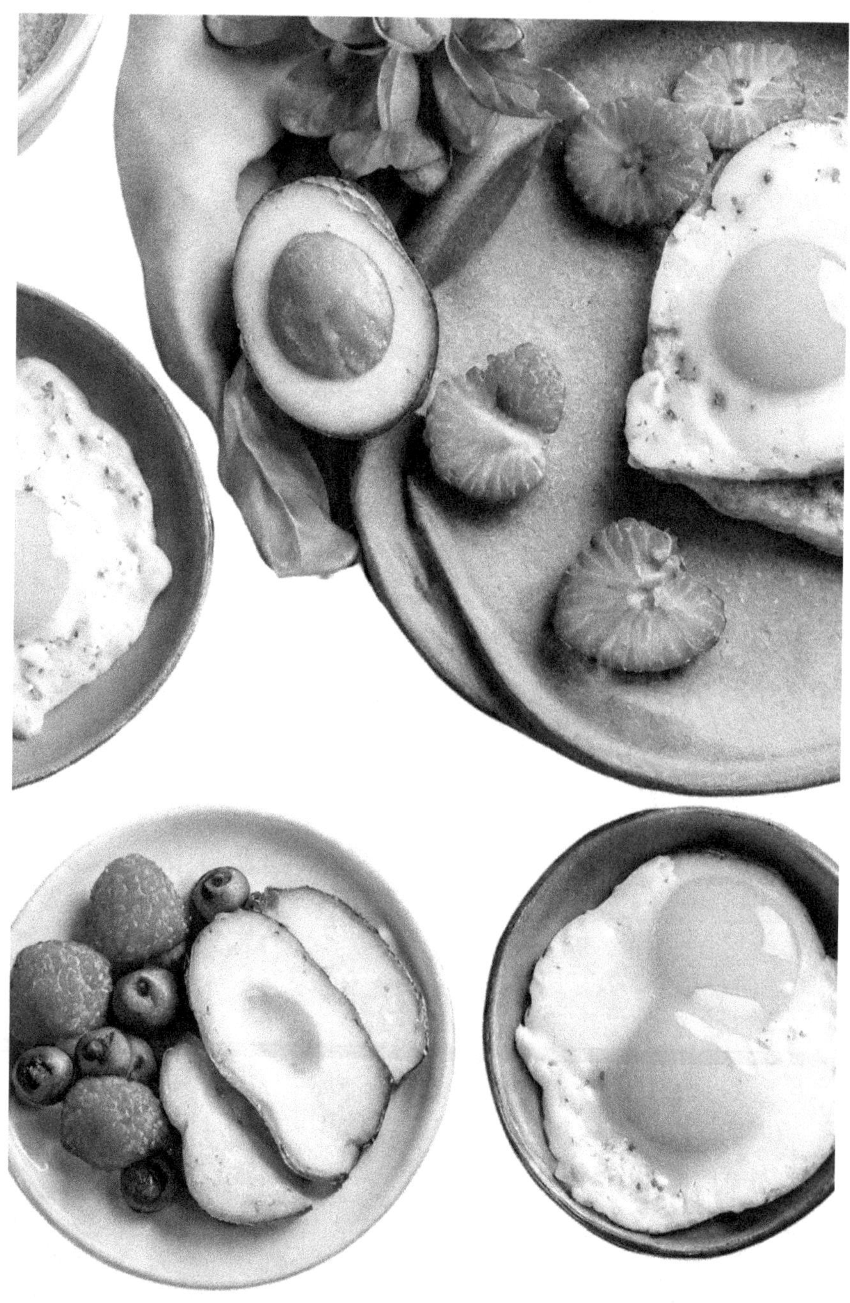

CHAPTER FOUR

Lunch Recipes

1. Quinoa Salad with Grilled Vegetables

- **Description:** A hearty and nutritious salad featuring protein-rich quinoa, colorful grilled vegetables, and a zesty vinaigrette for a satisfying and cancer-fighting lunch option.

- **Prep:** 15 minutes

- **Servings:** 4

- **Cooking Time:** 20 minutes

- **Nutritional Facts:** Approximately 300 calories per serving, high in fiber, vitamins, and antioxidants.

- **Ingredients:**

  - 1 cup quinoa, rinsed

  - 2 cups water or vegetable broth

- Assorted vegetables for grilling (such as bell peppers, zucchini, eggplant, and cherry tomatoes)

- 2 tablespoons olive oil

- Salt and pepper to taste

- For the vinaigrette: 1/4 cup extra virgin olive oil, 2 tablespoons balsamic vinegar, 1 teaspoon Dijon mustard, 1 clove garlic (minced), salt, and pepper

- **Instructions:**

1.   In a medium saucepan, combine quinoa and water or vegetable broth. Bring to a boil, then reduce heat to low, cover, and simmer for 15-20 minutes, or until quinoa is cooked and liquid is absorbed. Fluff with a fork and let cool.

2.   Preheat the grill to medium-high heat. Brush assorted vegetables with olive oil and season with salt and pepper.

3. Grill vegetables until tender and lightly charred, about 5-7 minutes per side. Remove from grill and let cool slightly.

4. In a small bowl, whisk together the ingredients for the vinaigrette until well combined.

5. In a large mixing bowl, combine cooked quinoa, grilled vegetables, and vinaigrette. Toss gently to coat.

6. Serve quinoa salad warm or chilled, garnished with fresh herbs if desired.

2. Salmon and Asparagus Foil Packets

- **Description:** A flavorful and nutritious meal featuring omega-3-rich salmon, vibrant asparagus, and aromatic herbs cooked in individual foil packets for easy cleanup and maximum flavor.

- **Prep:** 10 minutes

- **Servings:** 2

- **Cooking Time:** 20 minutes

- **Nutritional Facts:** Approximately 350 calories per serving, high in protein, omega-3 fatty acids, vitamins, and minerals.

- **Ingredients:**

  - 2 salmon fillets (about 6 ounces each)

  - 1 bunch asparagus, trimmed

  - 2 tablespoons olive oil

  - 2 cloves garlic, minced

  - 1 lemon, thinly sliced

  - Fresh herbs (such as dill, parsley, or thyme)

  - Salt and pepper to taste

- **Instructions:**

1. Preheat oven to 400°F (200°C). Cut two large pieces of aluminum foil.

2. Place each salmon fillet in the center of a piece of foil. Arrange asparagus spears around the salmon.

3. Drizzle olive oil over the salmon and asparagus. Sprinkle minced garlic, salt, and pepper over the top.

4. Place lemon slices and fresh herbs on top of the salmon.

5. Fold the edges of the foil over the salmon and vegetables to create a packet, sealing tightly.

6. Place foil packets on a baking sheet and bake in the preheated oven for 15-20 minutes, or until salmon is cooked through and asparagus is tender.

7. Carefully open the foil packets and transfer the salmon and asparagus to serving plates.

8. Serve immediately, garnished with additional fresh herbs and lemon wedges if desired.

3. Lentil and Vegetable Soup

- **Description:** A hearty and comforting soup featuring protein-packed lentils, an assortment of vegetables, and aromatic spices for a nourishing and immune-boosting lunch option.

- **Prep:** 15 minutes

- **Servings:** 6

- **Cooking Time:** 30 minutes

- **Nutritional Facts:** Approximately 250 calories per serving, high in fiber, protein, vitamins, and minerals.

- **Ingredients:**

  - 1 cup dried green or brown lentils, rinsed

  - 6 cups vegetable broth

  - 1 onion, chopped

  - 2 carrots, diced

  - 2 celery stalks, diced

  - 2 cloves garlic, minced

  - 1 teaspoon ground cumin

  - 1/2 teaspoon ground turmeric

  - 1/2 teaspoon smoked paprika

- Salt and pepper to taste

- Fresh parsley or cilantro for garnish

- **Instructions:**

1. In a large pot, combine lentils, vegetable broth, chopped onion, diced carrots, diced celery, minced garlic, ground cumin, ground turmeric, and smoked paprika. Season with salt and pepper to taste.

2. Bring the soup to a boil, then reduce heat to low and simmer for 20-25 minutes, or until lentils and vegetables are tender.

3. Taste and adjust seasoning if necessary.

4. Ladle soup into bowls and garnish with fresh parsley or cilantro.

5. Serve hot with crusty bread or whole-grain crackers.

4. Grilled Chicken Salad with Mixed Greens

- **Description:** A light and refreshing salad featuring grilled chicken breast, mixed greens, colorful vegetables, and a tangy vinaigrette for a satisfying and nutritious lunch option.

- **Prep:** 15 minutes

- **Servings:** 2

- **Cooking Time:** 15 minutes

- **Nutritional Facts:** Approximately 300 calories per serving, high in protein, vitamins, and antioxidants.

- **Ingredients:**

  - 2 boneless, skinless chicken breasts

  - 4 cups mixed greens (such as spinach, arugula, and romaine)

  - 1 cup cherry tomatoes, halved

  - 1/2 cucumber, sliced

- 1/4 red onion, thinly sliced

- 1/4 cup sliced almonds

- For the vinaigrette: 2 tablespoons extra virgin olive oil, 1 tablespoon balsamic vinegar, 1 teaspoon Dijon mustard, 1 teaspoon honey, salt, and pepper

- **Instructions:**

1. Preheat the grill or grill pan to medium-high heat. Season chicken breasts with salt and pepper.

2. Grill chicken breasts for 6-7 minutes per side, or until cooked through and no longer pink in the center. Remove from grill and let rest for a few minutes before slicing.

3. In a large mixing bowl, combine mixed greens, cherry tomatoes, sliced cucumber, and thinly sliced red onion.

4. In a small bowl, whisk together the ingredients for the vinaigrette until well combined.

5. Drizzle vinaigrette over the salad and toss gently to coat.

6. Divide salad mixture onto serving plates and top with sliced grilled chicken.

7. Sprinkle sliced almonds over the top.

8. Serve immediately, garnished with fresh herbs if desired.

5. Whole Grain Wrap with Hummus and Vegetables

- **Description:** A quick and satisfying lunch option featuring a whole grain wrap filled with creamy hummus, crunchy vegetables, and flavorful herbs for a delicious and nutritious meal on the go.

- **Prep:** 10 minutes

- **Servings:** 1

- **Cooking Time:** 0 minutes

- **Nutritional Facts:** Approximately 350 calories per serving, high in fiber, protein, vitamins, and minerals.

- **Ingredients:**

  - 1 whole grain wrap or tortilla

  - 2 tablespoons hummus

  - Assorted vegetables for filling (such as shredded carrots, cucumber slices, bell pepper strips, and leafy greens)

  - Fresh herbs (such as parsley, cilantro, or basil)

  - Salt and pepper to taste

- **Instructions:**

1. Lay the whole-grain wrap or tortilla on a flat surface.

2. Spread hummus evenly over the surface of the wrap.

3.   Arrange assorted vegetables and fresh herbs on top of the hummus.

4.   Season with salt and pepper to taste.

5.   Carefully roll up the wrap, tucking in the sides as you go.

6.   Slice the wrap in half diagonally and serve immediately, or wrap in foil or parchment paper for later.

6. Mediterranean Quinoa Salad

- **Description:** A vibrant and flavorful salad featuring protein-rich quinoa, fresh vegetables, tangy feta cheese, and briny olives tossed in a lemon-herb vinaigrette for a refreshing and satisfying lunch option.

- **Prep:** 15 minutes

- **Servings:** 4

- **Cooking Time:** 20 minutes

- **Nutritional Facts:** Approximately 300 calories per serving, high in fiber, protein, vitamins, and antioxidants.

- **Ingredients:**

  - 1 cup quinoa, rinsed

  - 2 cups water or vegetable broth

  - 1 cucumber, diced

  - 1-pint cherry tomatoes, halved

  - 1/4 cup red onion, finely chopped

  - 1/4 cup Kalamata olives, pitted and halved

  - 1/4 cup crumbled feta cheese

  - For the lemon-herb vinaigrette: 1/4 cup extra virgin olive oil, 2 tablespoons lemon juice, 1 teaspoon dried oregano, 1 teaspoon dried basil, salt, and pepper

- **Instructions:**

1.   In a medium saucepan, combine quinoa and water or vegetable broth. Bring to a boil, then reduce heat to low, cover, and simmer for 15-20 minutes, or until quinoa is cooked and liquid is absorbed. Fluff with a fork and let cool.

2.   In a large mixing bowl, combine cooked quinoa, diced cucumber, cherry tomatoes, finely chopped red onion, Kalamata olives, and crumbled feta cheese.

3.   In a small bowl, whisk together the ingredients for the lemon-herb vinaigrette until well combined.

4.   Pour vinaigrette over the quinoa salad and toss gently to coat.

5.   Serve quinoa salad chilled or at room temperature, garnished with fresh herbs if desired.

7. Veggie and Hummus Wrap

- **Description:** A nutritious and satisfying lunch wrap filled with creamy hummus and a variety of colorful vegetables for a flavorful and wholesome meal on the go.

- **Prep:** 10 minutes

- **Servings:** 1

- **Cooking Time:** 0 minutes

- **Nutritional Facts:** Approximately 250 calories per serving, high in fiber, vitamins, and minerals.

- **Ingredients:**

  - 1 whole grain wrap or tortilla

  - 2 tablespoons hummus

  - Assorted vegetables for filling (such as sliced cucumber, shredded carrots, bell pepper strips, and leafy greens)

  - Fresh herbs (such as cilantro or parsley)

  - Salt and pepper to taste

- **Instructions:**

1. Lay the whole-grain wrap or tortilla on a flat surface.

2.   Spread hummus evenly over the surface of the wrap.

3.   Arrange assorted vegetables and fresh herbs on top of the hummus.

4.   Season with salt and pepper to taste.

5.   Carefully roll up the wrap, tucking in the sides as you go.

6.   Slice the wrap in half diagonally and serve immediately, or wrap in foil or parchment paper for later.

8. Black Bean and Quinoa Stuffed Bell Peppers

- **Description:** Colorful bell peppers stuffed with protein-rich black beans, quinoa, vegetables, and savory spices for a hearty and nutritious lunch option that's packed with flavor.

- **Prep:** 20 minutes

- **Servings:** 4

- **Cooking Time:** 30 minutes

- **Nutritional Facts:** Approximately 300 calories per serving, high in fiber, protein, vitamins, and minerals.

- **Ingredients:**

  - 4 large bell peppers (any color), halved and seeds removed

  - 1 cup cooked quinoa

  - 1 can (15 ounces) black beans, drained and rinsed

  - 1 cup diced tomatoes

  - 1/2 cup corn kernels (fresh, frozen, or canned)

  - 1/4 cup chopped cilantro

  - 1 teaspoon ground cumin

  - 1 teaspoon chili powder

  - Salt and pepper to taste

- Optional toppings: avocado slices, shredded cheese, Greek yogurt or sour cream

- **Instructions:**

1. Preheat oven to 375°F (190°C). Arrange bell pepper halves in a baking dish.

2. In a large mixing bowl, combine cooked quinoa, black beans, diced tomatoes, corn kernels, chopped cilantro, ground cumin, chili powder, salt, and pepper. Stir until well combined.

3. Spoon quinoa and black bean mixture evenly into each bell pepper half, pressing down gently to pack the filling.

4. Cover the baking dish with foil and bake in the preheated oven for 25-30 minutes, or until bell peppers are tender.

5. Remove foil and bake for an additional 5 minutes, or until filling is heated through and the tops of peppers are slightly browned.

6.   Remove from oven and let cool slightly before serving.

7.   Serve stuffed bell peppers hot, garnished with optional toppings if desired.

9. Chickpea Salad with Lemon Tahini Dressing

- **Description:** A refreshing and protein-packed salad featuring chickpeas, crisp vegetables, and a creamy lemon tahini dressing for a light and satisfying lunch option.

- **Prep:** 15 minutes

- **Servings:** 4

- **Cooking Time:** 0 minutes

- **Nutritional Facts:** Approximately 250 calories per serving, high in fiber, protein, vitamins, and minerals.

- **Ingredients:**

- 2 cans (15 ounces each) chickpeas, drained and rinsed

- 1 cucumber, diced

- 1 bell pepper, diced

- 1/4 red onion, finely chopped

- 1/4 cup chopped parsley

- For the lemon tahini dressing: 1/4 cup tahini, 2 tablespoons lemon juice, 1 clove garlic (minced), 2 tablespoons water, salt, and pepper

- **Instructions:**

1. In a large mixing bowl, combine chickpeas, diced cucumber, diced bell pepper, finely chopped red onion, and chopped parsley.

2. In a small bowl, whisk together the ingredients for the lemon tahini dressing until smooth and creamy. If necessary, add more water to achieve the desired consistency.

3.   Pour dressing over the chickpea salad and toss gently to coat.

4.   Taste and adjust seasoning if necessary.

5.   Serve chickpea salad chilled or at room temperature, garnished with additional parsley if desired.

10. Tomato Basil Quinoa Soup

- **Description:** A comforting and flavorful soup featuring protein-rich quinoa, ripe tomatoes, fragrant basil, and aromatic spices for a nourishing and satisfying lunch option.

- **Prep:** 15 minutes

- **Servings:** 4

- **Cooking Time:** 30 minutes

- **Nutritional Facts:** Approximately 200 calories per serving, high in fiber, protein, vitamins, and antioxidants.

- **Ingredients:**

- 1 cup quinoa, rinsed

- 6 cups vegetable broth

- 4 cups chopped tomatoes (fresh or canned)

- 1 onion, chopped

- 2 cloves garlic, minced

- 1/4 cup chopped fresh basil

- 1 teaspoon dried oregano

- 1/2 teaspoon dried thyme

- Salt and pepper to taste

- **Instructions:**

1. In a large pot, combine quinoa, vegetable broth, chopped tomatoes, chopped onion, minced garlic, dried oregano, and dried thyme. Season with salt and pepper to taste.

2. Bring the soup to a boil, then reduce heat to low and simmer for 20-25 minutes, or until quinoa is cooked and flavors are well blended.

3.   Stir in chopped fresh basil and simmer for an additional 5 minutes.

4.   Taste and adjust seasoning if necessary.

5.   Serve tomato basil quinoa soup hot, garnished with additional fresh basil if desired.

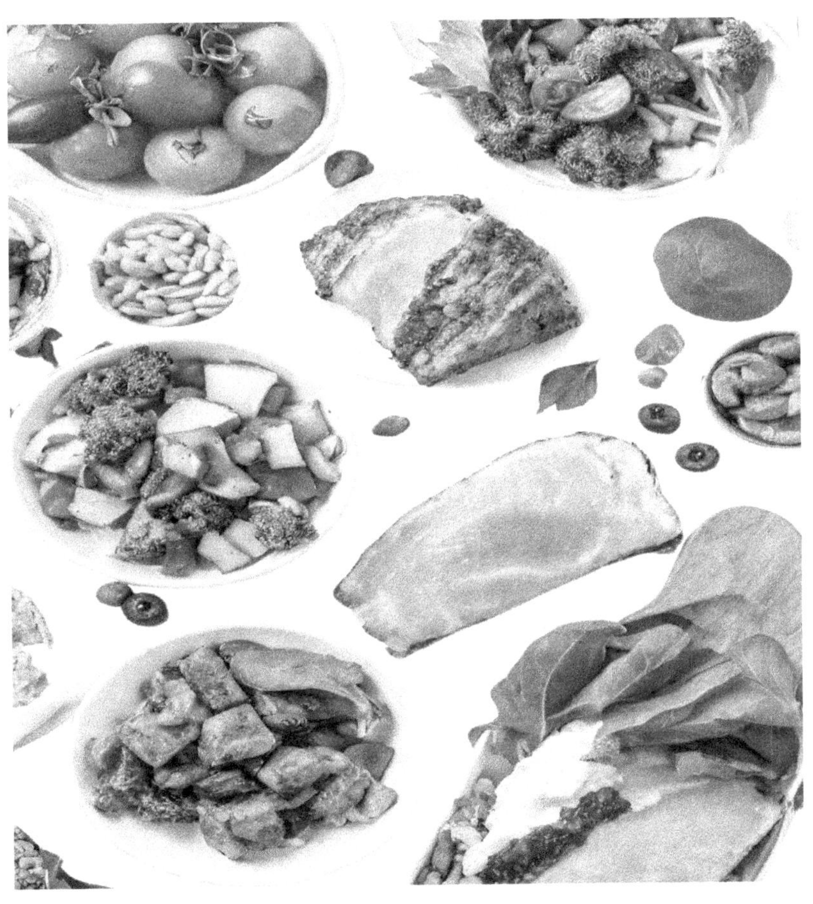

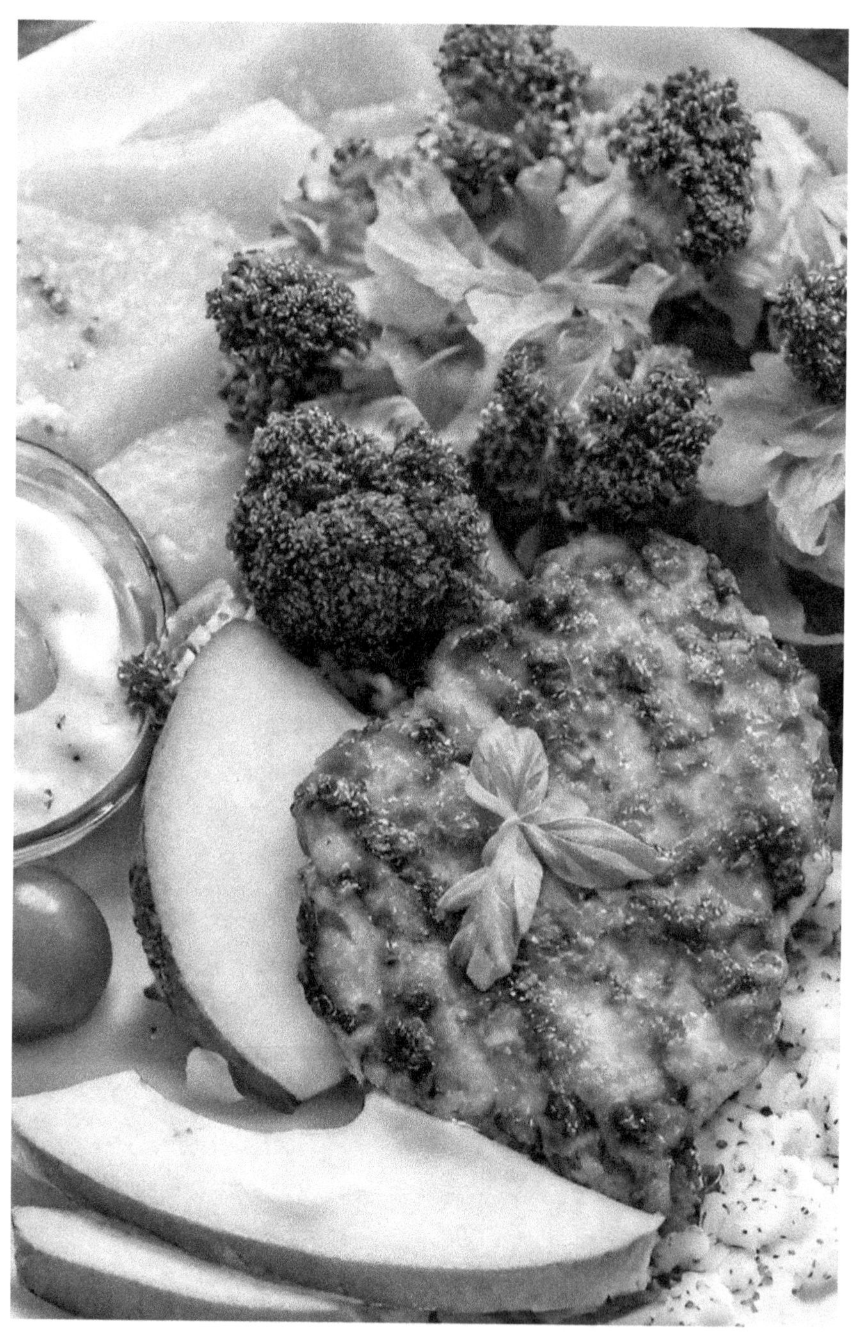

CHAPTER FIVE

Dinner Recipes

1. Grilled Salmon with Garlic Herb Butter

- **Description:** Succulent grilled salmon fillets topped with a flavorful garlic herb butter sauce for a delicious and nutritious dinner option rich in omega-3 fatty acids and antioxidants.

- **Prep:** 10 minutes

- **Servings:** 4

- **Cooking Time:** 10 minutes

- **Nutritional Facts:** Approximately 300 calories per serving, high in protein, omega-3 fatty acids, vitamins, and minerals.

- **Ingredients:**

  - 4 salmon fillets (about 6 ounces each)

- Salt and pepper to taste

- 4 tablespoons unsalted butter, softened

- 2 cloves garlic, minced

- 2 tablespoons chopped fresh herbs (such as parsley, dill, or chives)

- 1 lemon, sliced

- **Instructions:**

1. Preheat the grill to medium-high heat. Season salmon fillets with salt and pepper.

2. In a small bowl, mix softened butter, minced garlic, and chopped fresh herbs until well combined.

3. Place salmon fillets on the grill and cook for 4-5 minutes per side, or until fish is cooked through and flakes easily with a fork.

4. During the last minute of grilling, top each salmon fillet with a dollop of garlic herb butter.

5.   Remove salmon from the grill and transfer to serving plates.

6.   Garnish with lemon slices and serve immediately.

2. Veggie Stir-Fry with Tofu

- **Description:** A colorful and nutritious stir-fry featuring tofu and a variety of fresh vegetables tossed in a flavorful sauce for a satisfying and protein-rich dinner option.

- **Prep:** 15 minutes

- **Servings:** 4

- **Cooking Time:** 15 minutes

- **Nutritional Facts:** Approximately 250 calories per serving, high in protein, fiber, vitamins, and minerals.

- **Ingredients:**

    - 1 block (14 ounces) of firm tofu, drained and cubed

- 2 tablespoons soy sauce or tamari

- 1 tablespoon cornstarch

- 2 tablespoons sesame oil

- 2 cloves garlic, minced

- 1 tablespoon minced ginger

- Assorted vegetables for stir-fry (such as bell peppers, broccoli, carrots, snap peas)

- Cooked brown rice or quinoa for serving

- **Instructions:**

1.	In a small bowl, combine cubed tofu, soy sauce or tamari, and cornstarch. Toss until tofu is evenly coated.

2.	Heat sesame oil in a large skillet or wok over medium-high heat. Add minced garlic and minced ginger, and cook for 1 minute until fragrant.

3.	Add tofu to the skillet and cook, stirring occasionally, for 5-7 minutes, or until tofu is golden brown and crispy on the outside.

4.   Remove tofu from the skillet and set aside.

5.   In the same skillet, add additional sesame oil if needed and stir-fry assorted vegetables until crisp-tender, about 5 minutes.

6.   Return cooked tofu to the skillet and toss with the vegetables until heated through.

7.   Serve stir-fry over cooked brown rice or quinoa.

3. Roasted Vegetable Quinoa Bowl

- **Description:** A wholesome and satisfying bowl featuring roasted vegetables, protein-rich quinoa, and creamy avocado for a nutritious and flavorful dinner option.

- **Prep:** 15 minutes

- **Servings:** 4

- **Cooking Time:** 30 minutes

- **Nutritional Facts:** Approximately 300 calories per serving, high in fiber, protein, vitamins, and antioxidants.

- **Ingredients:**

  - 1 cup quinoa, rinsed

  - 2 cups water or vegetable broth

  - Assorted vegetables for roasting (such as sweet potatoes, Brussels sprouts, cauliflower, red onion)

  - 2 tablespoons olive oil

  - Salt and pepper to taste

  - 1 avocado, sliced

  - For the dressing: 1/4 cup extra virgin olive oil, 2 tablespoons balsamic vinegar, 1 teaspoon Dijon mustard, 1 teaspoon honey, salt, and pepper

- **Instructions:**

1. Preheat oven to 400°F (200°C). Arrange assorted vegetables on a baking sheet.

2.   Drizzle olive oil over the vegetables and season with salt and pepper. Toss to coat evenly.

3.   Roast vegetables in the preheated oven for 25-30 minutes or until tender and caramelized.

4.   In a medium saucepan, combine quinoa and water or vegetable broth. Bring to a boil, then reduce heat to low, cover, and simmer for 15-20 minutes, or until quinoa is cooked and liquid is absorbed. Fluff with a fork and let cool.

5.   In a small bowl, whisk together the ingredients for the dressing until well combined.

6.   To assemble the bowls, divide cooked quinoa among serving bowls. Top with roasted vegetables and sliced avocado.

7.   Drizzle with dressing and serve immediately.

4. Baked Chicken Breast with Roasted Vegetables

- **Description:** Tender and juicy baked chicken breast served with a medley of roasted vegetables for a wholesome and protein-packed dinner option that's easy to prepare and full of flavor.

- **Prep:** 15 minutes

- **Servings:** 4

- **Cooking Time:** 30 minutes

- **Nutritional Facts:** Approximately 250 calories per serving, high in protein, vitamins, and minerals.

- **Ingredients:**

  - 4 boneless, skinless chicken breasts

  - 2 tablespoons olive oil

  - 2 cloves garlic, minced

  - 1 teaspoon dried herbs (such as rosemary, thyme, or oregano)

- Assorted vegetables for roasting (such as bell peppers, zucchini, cherry tomatoes, red onion)

- Salt and pepper to taste

- **Instructions:**

1.	Preheat oven to 400°F (200°C). Line a baking sheet with parchment paper or aluminum foil.

2.	Place chicken breasts on the prepared baking sheet. Drizzle with olive oil and sprinkle minced garlic and dried herbs over the top. Season with salt and pepper.

3.	Arrange assorted vegetables around the chicken breasts on the baking sheet. Drizzle with olive oil and season with salt and pepper.

4.	Bake in the preheated oven for 25-30 minutes, or until chicken is cooked through and juices run clear.

5.	Remove from oven and let the chicken rest for a few minutes before slicing.

6.   Serve baked chicken breast with roasted vegetables hot, garnished with fresh herbs if desired.

5. Lentil and Vegetable Curry

- **Description:** A flavorful and hearty curry featuring protein-rich lentils, colorful vegetables, and aromatic spices for a satisfying and plant-based dinner option that's both nutritious and delicious.

- **Prep:** 15 minutes

- **Servings:** 4

- **Cooking Time:** 30 minutes

- **Nutritional Facts:** Approximately 300 calories per serving, high in fiber, protein, vitamins, and antioxidants.

- **Ingredients:**

  - 1 cup dried green or brown lentils, rinsed

  - 4 cups vegetable broth

  - 1 tablespoon olive oil

- 1 onion, chopped

- 2 cloves garlic, minced

- 1 tablespoon grated ginger

- 2 tablespoons curry powder

- 1 teaspoon ground turmeric

- 1 can (14 ounces) diced tomatoes

- Assorted vegetables (such as cauliflower, carrots, bell peppers, peas)

- Salt and pepper to taste

- **Instructions:**

1. In a large pot, heat olive oil over medium heat. Add chopped onion and cook until softened about 5 minutes.

2. Add minced garlic, grated ginger, curry powder, and ground turmeric to the pot. Cook for 1-2 minutes until fragrant.

3.   Stir in dried lentils, vegetable broth, and diced tomatoes. Bring to a boil, then reduce heat to low, cover, and simmer for 20-25 minutes, or until lentils are tender.

4.   Add assorted vegetables to the pot and simmer for an additional 5-7 minutes, or until vegetables are cooked to your liking.

5.   Season with salt and pepper to taste.

6.   Serve lentil and vegetable curry hot, garnished with fresh cilantro if desired, and accompanied by cooked brown rice or naan bread.

6. Grilled Veggie and Chickpea Buddha Bowl

- **Description:** A nourishing and vibrant Buddha bowl featuring grilled vegetables, protein-packed chickpeas, creamy avocado, and a tangy tahini dressing for a wholesome and satisfying dinner option.

- **Prep:** 20 minutes

- **Servings:** 4

- **Cooking Time:** 20 minutes

- **Nutritional Facts:** Approximately 350 calories per serving, high in fiber, protein, vitamins, and healthy fats.

- **Ingredients:**

  - 1 can (15 ounces) chickpeas, drained and rinsed

  - 2 tablespoons olive oil

  - 1 teaspoon ground cumin

  - 1 teaspoon smoked paprika

  - Assorted vegetables for grilling (such as zucchini, eggplant, bell peppers, red onion)

  - 2 cups cooked quinoa or brown rice

  - 1 avocado, sliced

  - For the tahini dressing: 1/4 cup tahini, 2 tablespoons lemon juice, 1 clove garlic (minced), 2 tablespoons water, salt, and pepper

- **Instructions:**

1. Preheat the grill to medium-high heat.

2. In a large mixing bowl, toss drained and rinsed chickpeas with olive oil, ground cumin, smoked paprika, salt, and pepper.

3. Thread assorted vegetables onto skewers or grill baskets.

4. Grill chickpeas and vegetables for 8-10 minutes, turning occasionally, until chickpeas are crispy and vegetables are tender and charred.

5. In a small bowl, whisk together the ingredients for the tahini dressing until smooth and creamy. If necessary, add more water to achieve the desired consistency.

6. To assemble the Buddha bowls, divide cooked quinoa or brown rice among serving bowls. Top with grilled vegetables, chickpeas, and sliced avocado.

7.   Drizzle with tahini dressing and serve immediately.

7. Stuffed Bell Peppers with Turkey and Quinoa

- **Description:** Colorful bell peppers stuffed with lean ground turkey, protein-rich quinoa, and flavorful spices for a wholesome and satisfying dinner option that's both nutritious and delicious.

- **Prep:** 20 minutes

- **Servings:** 4

- **Cooking Time:** 40 minutes

- **Nutritional Facts:** Approximately 300 calories per serving, high in protein, fiber, vitamins, and minerals.

- **Ingredients:**

  - 4 large bell peppers (any color), halved and seeds removed

  - 1 pound lean ground turkey

- 1 cup cooked quinoa

- 1 can (14 ounces) diced tomatoes, drained

- 1/2 cup diced onion

- 2 cloves garlic, minced

- 1 teaspoon dried oregano

- 1 teaspoon dried basil

- Salt and pepper to taste

- **Instructions:**

1.   Preheat oven to 375°F (190°C). Arrange bell pepper halves in a baking dish.

2.   In a large skillet, cook ground turkey over medium heat until browned and cooked, breaking it apart with a spoon.

3.   Add diced onion and minced garlic to the skillet with the turkey, and cook for an additional 2-3 minutes until the onion is softened.

4.   Stir in cooked quinoa, diced tomatoes, dried oregano, dried basil, salt, and pepper. Cook for 2-3 minutes until heated through and well combined.

5.   Spoon the turkey and quinoa mixture evenly into each bell pepper half, pressing down gently to pack the filling.

6.   Cover the baking dish with foil and bake in the preheated oven for 30-35 minutes, or until bell peppers are tender.

7.   Remove foil and bake for an additional 5 minutes, or until the tops of the peppers are slightly browned.

8.   Serve stuffed bell peppers hot, garnished with fresh herbs if desired.

8. Eggplant and Chickpea Curry

- **Description:** A fragrant and flavorful curry featuring tender eggplant, protein-rich chickpeas, and aromatic spices for a comforting and nutritious dinner option that's perfect served with rice or naan bread.

- **Prep:** 20 minutes

- **Servings:** 4

- **Cooking Time:** 30 minutes

- **Nutritional Facts:** Approximately 250 calories per serving, high in fiber, protein, vitamins, and antioxidants.

- **Ingredients:**

  - 1 large eggplant, diced

  - 1 can (15 ounces) chickpeas, drained and rinsed

  - 1 onion, chopped

  - 2 cloves garlic, minced

  - 1 tablespoon grated ginger

  - 2 tablespoons curry powder

  - 1 teaspoon ground turmeric

  - 1 can (14 ounces) diced tomatoes

- 1 can (14 ounces) coconut milk

- Salt and pepper to taste

- **Instructions:**

1. Heat olive oil in a large pot or skillet over medium heat. Add chopped onion and cook until softened about 5 minutes.

2. Add minced garlic, grated ginger, curry powder, and ground turmeric to the pot. Cook for 1-2 minutes until fragrant.

3. Add diced eggplant to the pot and cook for 5-7 minutes until slightly softened.

4. Stir in drained and rinsed chickpeas, diced tomatoes, and coconut milk. Bring to a simmer and cook for 15-20 minutes, stirring occasionally, until the eggplant is tender and the flavors are well blended.

5. Season with salt and pepper to taste.

6.   Serve eggplant and chickpea curry hot, garnished with fresh cilantro if desired, and accompanied by cooked brown rice or naan bread.

9. Spinach and Mushroom Stuffed Chicken Breast

- **Description:** Juicy chicken breasts stuffed with a flavorful mixture of spinach, mushrooms, and cheese for an elegant and satisfying dinner option that's perfect for entertaining or a special weeknight meal.

- **Prep:** 20 minutes

- **Servings:** 4

- **Cooking Time:** 30 minutes

- **Nutritional Facts:** Approximately 300 calories per serving, high in protein, vitamins, and minerals.

- **Ingredients:**

    - 4 boneless, skinless chicken breasts

- Salt and pepper to taste

- 1 tablespoon olive oil

- 2 cups fresh spinach, chopped

- 1 cup mushrooms, finely chopped

- 2 cloves garlic, minced

- 1/2 cup shredded mozzarella cheese

- 1/4 cup grated Parmesan cheese

- **Instructions:**

1. Preheat oven to 375°F (190°C). Line a baking dish with parchment paper or aluminum foil.

2. Using a sharp knife, make a horizontal slit along the side of each chicken breast to create a pocket for stuffing. Be careful not to cut all the way through.

3. Season the inside of each chicken breast with salt and pepper.

4. In a skillet, heat olive oil over medium heat. Add chopped spinach, mushrooms, and minced garlic. Cook

for 3-4 minutes until spinach is wilted and mushrooms are tender. Remove from heat and let cool slightly.

5.   Stir shredded mozzarella cheese and grated Parmesan cheese into the spinach and mushroom mixture.

6.   Stuff each chicken breast with the spinach and mushroom mixture, pressing down gently to pack the filling.

7.   Place stuffed chicken breasts in the prepared baking dish.

8.   Bake in the preheated oven for 25-30 minutes, or until chicken is cooked through and juices run clear.

9.   Remove from oven and let the chicken rest for a few minutes before serving.

10. Spaghetti Squash with Turkey Bolognese

- **Description:** A lighter twist on classic spaghetti Bolognese featuring spaghetti squash noodles topped with a savory turkey and tomato sauce for a flavorful and low-carb dinner option that's hearty and satisfying.

- **Prep:** 20 minutes

- **Servings:** 4

- **Cooking Time:** 1 hour

- **Nutritional Facts:** Approximately 300 calories per serving, low in carbohydrates, high in protein, vitamins, and minerals.

- **Ingredients:**

  - 1 large spaghetti squash

  - 1 tablespoon olive oil

  - 1 pound lean ground turkey

  - 1 onion, chopped

  - 2 cloves garlic, minced

  - 1 can (14 ounces) diced tomatoes

  - 1 can (6 ounces) tomato paste

- 1 teaspoon dried oregano

- 1 teaspoon dried basil

- Salt and pepper to taste

- **Instructions:**

1.   Preheat oven to 375°F (190°C). Cut spaghetti squash in half lengthwise and scoop out the seeds.

2.   Place squash halves cut side down on a baking sheet lined with parchment paper or aluminum foil. Bake in the preheated oven for 40-45 minutes, or until squash is tender and easily pierced with a fork.

3.   While the squash is baking, heat olive oil in a large skillet over medium heat. Add chopped onion and cook until softened about 5 minutes.

4.   Add minced garlic to the skillet and cook for 1-2 minutes until fragrant.

5.   Add ground turkey to the skillet and cook until browned and cooked, breaking it apart with a spoon.

6.	Stir in diced tomatoes, tomato paste, dried oregano, dried basil, salt, and pepper. Simmer for 10-15 minutes, stirring occasionally, until sauce is thickened and flavors are well blended.

7.	Once the squash is cooked, use a fork to scrape the flesh into strands, creating "noodles."

8.	Divide spaghetti squash noodles among serving plates and top with turkey Bolognese sauce.

9.	Serve hot, garnished with grated Parmesan cheese and fresh basil if desired.

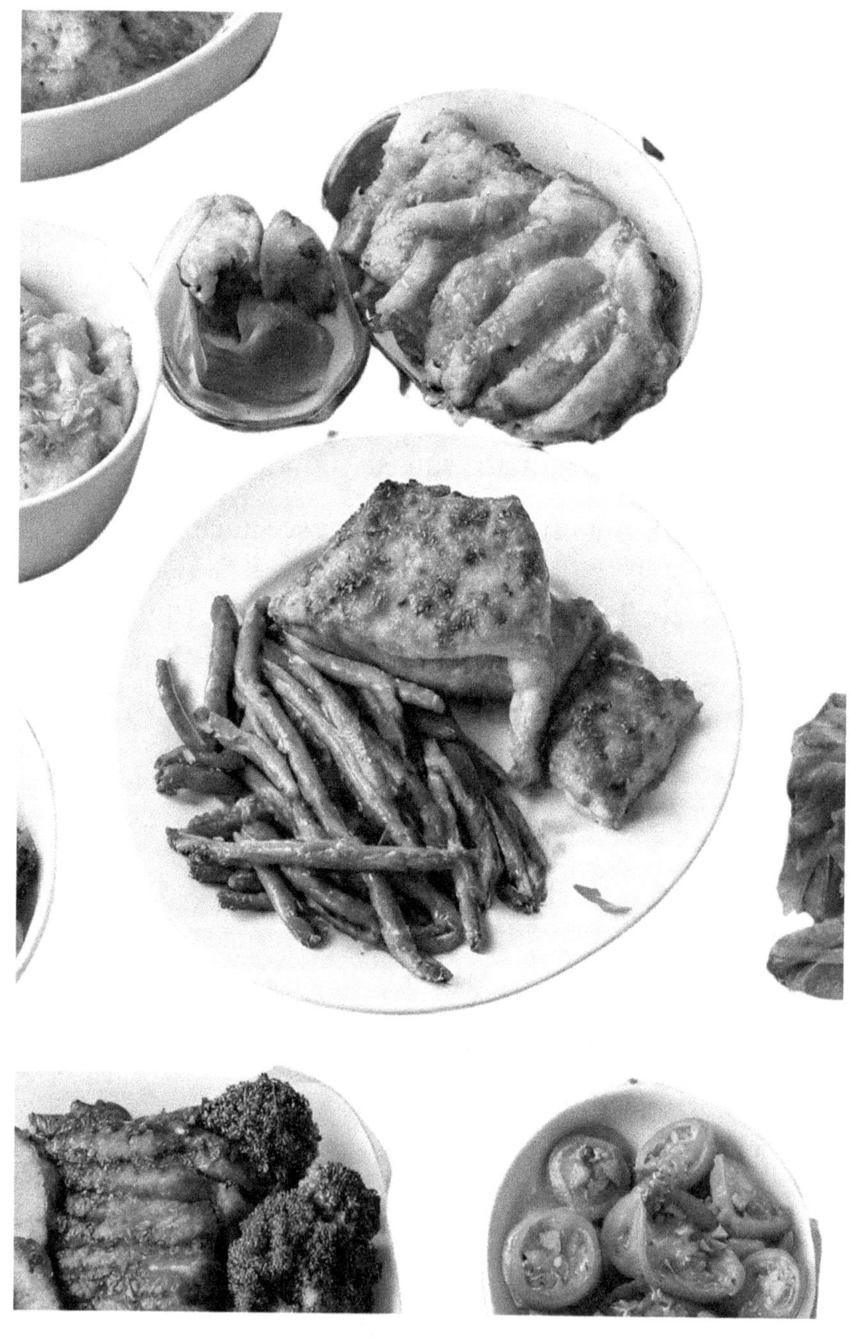

Snacks And Appetizers Recipes

1. Guacamole with Veggie Sticks

- **Description:** Creamy and flavorful guacamole served with a variety of colorful vegetable sticks for a nutritious and satisfying snack or appetizer.

- **Prep:** 10 minutes

- **Servings:** 4

- **Cooking Time:** 0 minutes

- **Nutritional Facts:** Approximately 150 calories per serving, high in healthy fats, fiber, vitamins, and minerals.

- **Ingredients:**

  - 2 ripe avocados

  - 1 lime, juiced

  - 1/4 cup diced red onion

- 1 small tomato, diced

- 1/4 cup chopped cilantro

- Salt and pepper to taste

- Assorted vegetable sticks (such as carrot, cucumber, bell pepper, celery)

- **Instructions:**

1. Cut avocados in half, remove pits, and scoop the flesh into a bowl.

2. Mash the avocado with a fork until smooth or chunky, depending on your preference.

3. Add lime juice, diced red onion, diced tomato, and chopped cilantro to the mashed avocado. Mix well to combine.

4. Season with salt and pepper to taste.

5. Serve guacamole with assorted vegetable sticks for dipping.

2. Greek Yogurt Dip with Whole Grain Crackers

- **Description:** Creamy and tangy Greek yogurt dip flavored with herbs and spices, served with whole grain crackers for a satisfying and protein-rich snack.

- **Prep:** 5 minutes

- **Servings:** 4

- **Cooking Time:** 0 minutes

- **Nutritional Facts:** Approximately 100 calories per serving, high in protein, calcium, and probiotics.

- **Ingredients:**

  - 1 cup Greek yogurt

  - 1 tablespoon chopped fresh dill

  - 1 tablespoon chopped fresh parsley

  - 1 clove garlic, minced

  - 1/2 teaspoon lemon zest

- Salt and pepper to taste

- Whole grain crackers for serving

- **Instructions:**

1. Mix Greek yogurt, chopped fresh dill, chopped fresh parsley, minced garlic, and lemon zest until well combined.

2. Season with salt and pepper to taste.

3. Serve Greek yogurt dip with whole grain crackers for dipping.

3. Hummus Hummus-stuffed cucumber Cups

- **Description:** Crisp cucumber cups filled with creamy hummus and garnished with fresh herbs for a refreshing and nutritious snack or appetizer.

- **Prep:** 15 minutes

- **Servings:** 4

- **Cooking Time:** 0 minutes

- **Nutritional Facts:** Approximately 100 calories per serving, high in fiber, protein, vitamins, and minerals.

- **Ingredients:**

  - 2 large cucumbers

  - 1/2 cup hummus

  - Fresh parsley or dill for garnish

- **Instructions:**

1. Cut cucumbers into thick slices, about 2 inches thick.

2. Use a small spoon or melon baller to scoop out the seeds from the center of each cucumber slice, creating a cup shape.

3. Fill each cucumber cup with a spoonful of hummus.

4. Garnish with fresh parsley or dill.

5. Serve immediately or refrigerate until ready to serve.

4. Caprese Skewers

- **Description:** Bite-sized skewers featuring cherry tomatoes, fresh mozzarella balls, and basil leaves drizzled with balsamic glaze for a simple and elegant snack or appetizer.

- **Prep:** 10 minutes

- **Servings:** 4

- **Cooking Time:** 0 minutes

- **Nutritional Facts:** Approximately 100 calories per serving, high in protein, calcium, and antioxidants.

- **Ingredients:**

  - Cherry tomatoes

  - Fresh mozzarella balls (bocconcini)

  - Fresh basil leaves

  - Balsamic glaze

- **Instructions:**

1.   Thread cherry tomatoes, fresh mozzarella balls, and fresh basil leaves onto skewers, alternating the ingredients.

2.   Arrange skewers on a serving platter.

3.   Drizzle with balsamic glaze just before serving.

4.   Serve immediately.

5. Almond Butter and Banana Slices

- **Description:** Creamy almond butter spread onto banana slices for a delicious and energizing snack loaded with healthy fats, protein, and potassium.

- **Prep:** 5 minutes

- **Servings:** 2

- **Cooking Time:** 0 minutes

- **Nutritional Facts:** Approximately 200 calories per serving, high in healthy fats, protein, fiber, and potassium.

- **Ingredients:**

  - 1 ripe banana, sliced

- 2 tablespoons almond butter

- **Instructions:**

1. Spread almond butter onto banana slices.

2. Arrange on a plate and serve immediately.

6. Quinoa Stuffed Mini Bell Peppers

- **Description:** Colorful mini bell peppers stuffed with quinoa salad for a flavorful and nutritious snack or appetizer that's packed with protein, fiber, and vitamins.

- **Prep:** 20 minutes

- **Servings:** 4

- **Cooking Time:** 0 minutes

- **Nutritional Facts:** Approximately 150 calories per serving, high in protein, fiber, vitamins, and minerals.

- **Ingredients:**

- 12 mini bell peppers, halved and seeds removed

- 1 cup cooked quinoa

- 1/4 cup diced cucumber

- 1/4 cup diced tomatoes

- 2 tablespoons chopped fresh parsley

- 1 tablespoon lemon juice

- Salt and pepper to taste

- **Instructions:**

1. In a bowl, combine cooked quinoa, diced cucumber, diced tomatoes, chopped fresh parsley, lemon juice, salt, and pepper. Mix well.

2. Fill each mini bell pepper half with a spoonful of quinoa salad.

3. Arrange stuffed mini bell peppers on a serving platter.

4.   Serve immediately or refrigerate until ready to serve.

7. Kale Chips

- **Description:** Crispy and flavorful kale chips seasoned with olive oil, salt, and nutritional yeast for a healthy and addictive snack that's rich in vitamins, minerals, and antioxidants.

- **Prep:** 10 minutes

- **Servings:** 4

- **Cooking Time:** 20 minutes

- **Nutritional Facts:** Approximately 100 calories per serving, high in fiber, vitamins, and antioxidants.

- **Ingredients:**

  - 1 bunch of kale, stems removed and torn into bite-sized pieces

  - 1 tablespoon olive oil

  - 1 tablespoon nutritional yeast

- Salt to taste

- **Instructions:**

1. Preheat oven to 275°F (135°C). Line a baking sheet with parchment paper.

2. In a large bowl, toss kale pieces with olive oil until evenly coated.

3. Sprinkle nutritional yeast and salt over the kale, and toss again to coat.

4. Spread kale pieces in a single layer on the prepared baking sheet.

5. Bake in the preheated oven for 20-25 minutes, or until kale is crisp and edges are slightly browned.

6. Remove from oven and let kale chips cool completely before serving.

8. Berry and Almond Yogurt Parfait

- **Description:** Layers of creamy yogurt, fresh berries, and crunchy almonds for a delicious and nutritious parfait that's perfect for breakfast or snack time.

- **Prep:** 10 minutes

- **Servings:** 2

- **Cooking Time:** 0 minutes

- **Nutritional Facts:** Approximately 200 calories per serving, high in protein, fiber, vitamins, and antioxidants.

- **Ingredients:**

  - 1 cup Greek yogurt

  - 1/2 cup fresh berries (such as strawberries, blueberries, raspberries)

  - 1/4 cup almonds, chopped

  - Honey or maple syrup for drizzling (optional)

- **Instructions:**

1. In serving glasses or bowls, layer Greek yogurt, fresh berries, and chopped almonds.

2.   Repeat layers until ingredients are used up.

3.   Drizzle with honey or maple syrup if desired.

4.   Serve berry and almond yogurt parfait immediately.

9. Spinach and Feta Stuffed Mushrooms

- **Description:** Tender mushroom caps filled with a savory mixture of spinach, feta cheese, and herbs for a flavorful and satisfying appetizer that's low in calories and high in nutrients.

- **Prep:** 15 minutes

- **Servings:** 4

- **Cooking Time:** 20 minutes

- **Nutritional Facts:** Approximately 100 calories per serving, high in protein, vitamins, and minerals.

- **Ingredients:**

  - 12 large mushrooms, stems removed and caps cleaned

  - 2 cups fresh spinach, chopped

- 1/4 cup crumbled feta cheese

- 1 clove garlic, minced

- 1 tablespoon olive oil

- Salt and pepper to taste

- **Instructions:**

1. Preheat oven to 375°F (190°C). Line a baking sheet with parchment paper.

2. In a skillet, heat olive oil over medium heat. Add minced garlic and chopped spinach, and cook until spinach is wilted, about 2-3 minutes.

3. Remove skillet from heat and stir in crumbled feta cheese. Season with salt and pepper to taste.

4. Spoon spinach and feta mixture into each mushroom cap, pressing down gently to pack the filling.

5. Place stuffed mushrooms on the prepared baking sheet.

6. Bake in the preheated oven for 15-20 minutes, or until mushrooms are tender and filling is heated through.

7. Serve spinach and feta stuffed mushrooms hot, garnished with fresh herbs if desired.

10. Smoked Salmon Cucumber Bites

- **Description:** Crisp cucumber slices topped with creamy herbed cream cheese and smoked salmon for an elegant and flavorful appetizer that's perfect for parties or gatherings.

- **Prep:** 15 minutes

- **Servings:** 4

- **Cooking Time:** 0 minutes

- **Nutritional Facts:** Approximately 150 calories per serving, high in protein, omega-3 fatty acids, vitamins, and minerals.

- **Ingredients:**

    - 1 English cucumber, sliced

- 4 ounces smoked salmon, sliced

- 1/4 cup cream cheese, softened

- 1 tablespoon chopped fresh dill

- 1 teaspoon lemon zest

- Salt and pepper to taste

- **Instructions:**

1. In a small bowl, mix softened cream cheese, chopped fresh dill, lemon zest, salt, and pepper until well combined.

2. Spread a thin layer of herbed cream cheese onto each cucumber slice.

3. Top with a slice of smoked salmon.

4. Arrange smoked salmon cucumber bites on a serving platter.

5. Serve immediately or refrigerate until ready to serve.

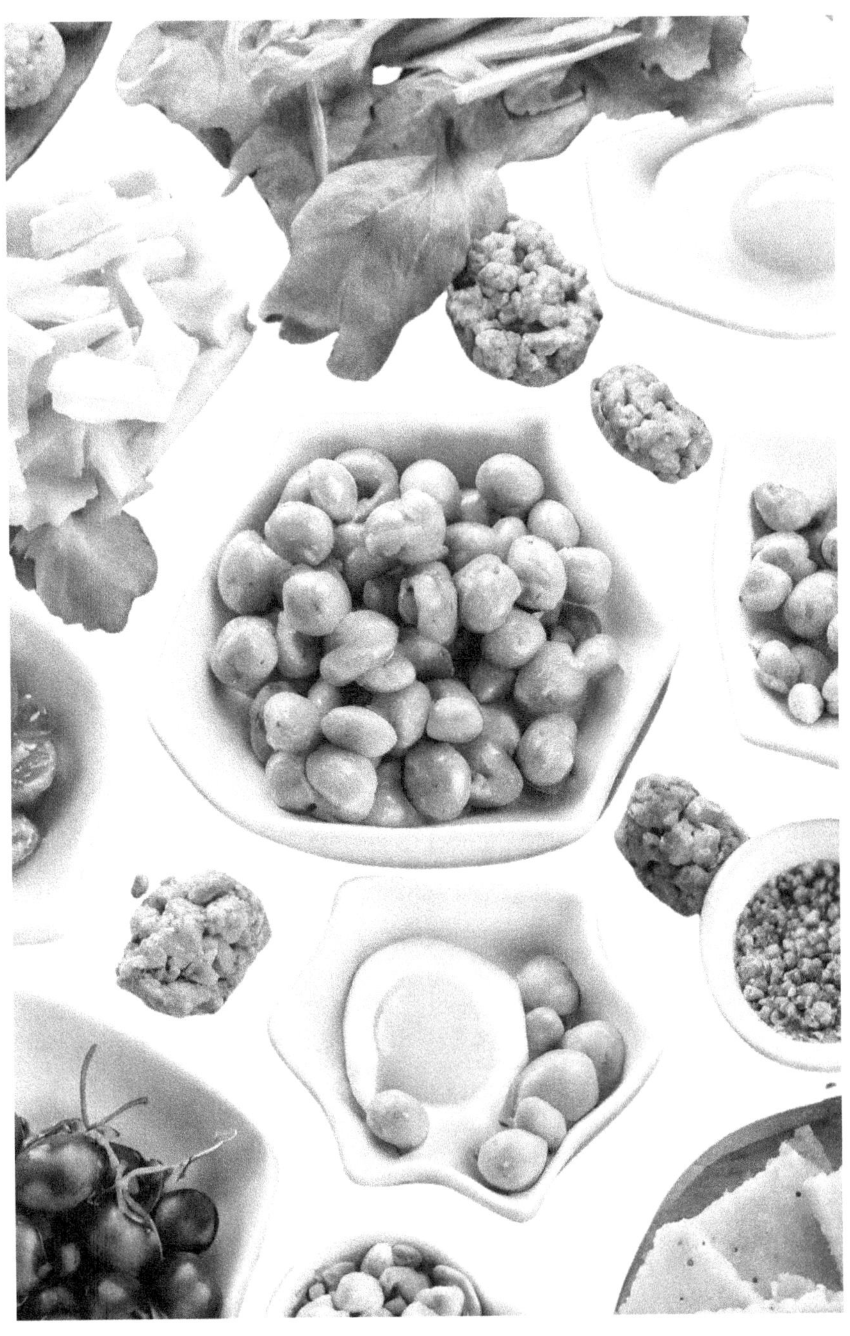

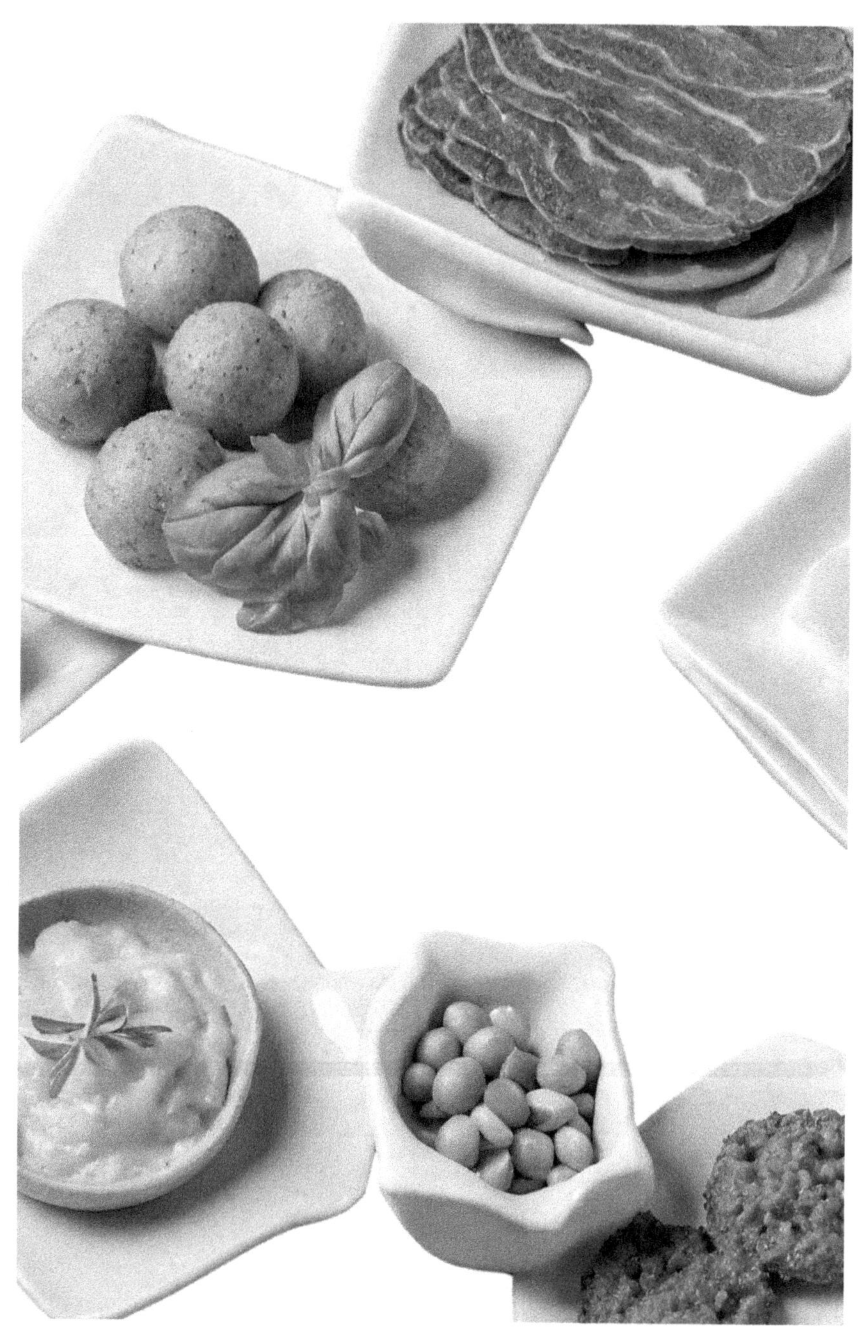

CHAPTER SEVEN

Smoothies and Juices Packed with Antioxidants

51. Green Detox Smoothie

- **Description:** Refreshing and cleansing green smoothie packed with nutrient-rich ingredients to support detoxification and overall health.

- **Prep:** 5 minutes

- **Servings:** 2

- **Cooking Time:** 0 minutes

- **Nutritional Facts:** Approximately 150 calories per serving, high in fiber, vitamins, minerals, and antioxidants.

- **Ingredients:**

  - 2 cups spinach

  - 1 cucumber, peeled and chopped

- 1 green apple, cored and chopped

- 1/2 lemon, juiced

- 1-inch piece of ginger, peeled

- 1 cup coconut water or water

- Ice cubes (optional)

- **Instructions:**

1. Place spinach, cucumber, green apple, lemon juice, ginger, and coconut water (or water) in a blender.

2. Blend until smooth and creamy.

3. If desired, add ice cubes and blend again until well incorporated.

4. Pour into glasses and serve immediately.

2. Berry Blast Smoothie

- **Description:** Vibrant and delicious berry smoothie loaded with antioxidants and vitamins to support immune health and fight inflammation.

- **Prep:** 5 minutes

- **Servings:** 2

- **Cooking Time:** 0 minutes

- **Nutritional Facts:** Approximately 200 calories per serving, high in fiber, vitamins, minerals, and antioxidants.

- **Ingredients:**

  - 1 cup mixed berries (such as strawberries, blueberries, or raspberries)

  - 1/2 banana, frozen

  - 1/2 cup Greek yogurt

  - 1 tablespoon chia seeds

  - 1 cup almond milk or other milk of choice

  - Honey or maple syrup to taste (optional)

- **Instructions:**

1. Place mixed berries, frozen banana, Greek yogurt, chia seeds, almond milk, and sweetener (if using) in a blender.

2.   Blend until smooth and creamy.

3.   Taste and adjust sweetness if necessary.

4.   Pour into glasses and serve immediately.

3. Tropical Turmeric Smoothie

- **Description:** Bright and tropical smoothie with a hint of turmeric, known for its anti-inflammatory properties, to support overall wellness.

- **Prep:** 5 minutes

- **Servings:** 2

- **Cooking Time:** 0 minutes

- **Nutritional Facts:** Approximately 180 calories per serving, high in fiber, vitamins, minerals, and antioxidants.

- **Ingredients:**

    - 1 cup frozen pineapple chunks

    - 1/2 cup frozen mango chunks

    - 1/2 banana

- 1/2 teaspoon ground turmeric

- 1/2 teaspoon ground ginger

- 1 cup coconut water or water

- **Instructions:**

1. Place frozen pineapple chunks, frozen mango chunks, banana, turmeric, ginger, and coconut water (or water) in a blender.

2. Blend until smooth and creamy.

3. If the smoothie is too thick, add more liquid as needed and blend again until the desired consistency is reached.

4. Pour into glasses and serve immediately.

4. Citrus Carrot Juice

- **Description:** Bright and zesty juice featuring citrus fruits and carrots for a refreshing and immune-boosting beverage.

- **Prep:** 10 minutes

- **Servings:** 2

- **Cooking Time:** 0 minutes

- **Nutritional Facts:** Approximately 120 calories per serving, high in vitamin C, beta-carotene, and antioxidants.

- **Ingredients:**

  - 3 oranges, peeled and segmented

  - 2 carrots, peeled and chopped

  - 1 lemon, peeled and segmented

  - 1-inch piece of ginger, peeled

- **Instructions:**

1. Pass oranges, carrots, lemon, and ginger through a juicer.

2. Stir the juice well to combine.

3. Pour into glasses and serve immediately over ice if desired.

5. Green Goddess Juice

- **Description:** Nourishing green juice loaded with leafy greens and refreshing herbs for a rejuvenating and cleansing beverage.

- **Prep:** 10 minutes

- **Servings:** 2

- **Cooking Time:** 0 minutes

- **Nutritional Facts:** Approximately 100 calories per serving, high in vitamins, minerals, and antioxidants.

- **Ingredients:**

  - 2 cups spinach

  - 1 cucumber, peeled

  - 1 green apple, cored

  - 1/2 cup fresh parsley leaves

  - 1/2 lemon, peeled

- **Instructions:**

1.   Pass spinach, cucumber, green apple, parsley, and lemon through a juicer.

2.   Stir the juice well to combine.

3.   Pour into glasses and serve immediately over ice if desired.

6. Beet Berry Detox Juice

- **Description:** Cleansing and vibrant juice featuring beets and berries for a detoxifying and antioxidant-rich beverage.

- **Prep:** 15 minutes

- **Servings:** 2

- **Cooking Time:** 0 minutes

- **Nutritional Facts:** Approximately 150 calories per serving, high in fiber, vitamins, minerals, and antioxidants.

- **Ingredients:**

  - 1 medium beet, peeled and chopped

- 1 cup mixed berries (such as strawberries, raspberries, blueberries)

- 1/2 lemon, peeled

- 1-inch piece of ginger, peeled

- **Instructions:**

1. Pass beet, mixed berries, lemon, and ginger through a juicer.

2. Stir the juice well to combine.

3. Pour into glasses and serve immediately over ice if desired.

7. Mango Ginger Turmeric Smoothie

- **Description:** Creamy and tropical smoothie with a kick of ginger and turmeric for a refreshing and anti-inflammatory beverage.

- **Prep:** 5 minutes

- **Servings:** 2

- **Cooking Time:** 0 minutes

- **Nutritional Facts:** Approximately 200 calories per serving, high in fiber, vitamins, minerals, and antioxidants.

- **Ingredients:**

  - 1 ripe mango, peeled and chopped

  - 1/2 banana, frozen

  - 1 cup coconut water or water

  - 1/2 teaspoon ground turmeric

  - 1/2 teaspoon grated ginger

- **Instructions:**

1. Place chopped mango, frozen banana, coconut water (or water), turmeric, and grated ginger in a blender.

2. Blend until smooth and creamy.

3. If the smoothie is too thick, add more liquid as needed and blend again until the desired consistency is reached.

4. Pour into glasses and serve immediately.

8. Blueberry Kale Smoothie

- **Description:** Nutrient-packed smoothie featuring blueberries and kale for a delicious and antioxidant-rich beverage.

- **Prep:** 5 minutes

- **Servings:** 2

- **Cooking Time:** 0 minutes

- **Nutritional Facts:** Approximately 150 calories per serving, high in fiber, vitamins, minerals, and antioxidants.

- **Ingredients:**

  - 1 cup frozen blueberries

  - 1 cup kale leaves, stemmed

  - 1/2 banana

  - 1 tablespoon almond butter

  - 1 cup almond milk or other milk of choice

- **Instructions:**

1.   Place frozen blueberries, kale leaves, banana, almond butter, and almond milk in a blender.

2.   Blend until smooth and creamy.

3.   If the smoothie is too thick, add more liquid as needed and blend again until the desired consistency is reached.

4.   Pour into glasses and serve immediately.

9. Pineapple Cucumber Mint Juice

- **Description:** Refreshing and hydrating juice featuring pineapple, cucumber, and mint for a cooling and revitalizing beverage.

- **Prep:** 10 minutes

- **Servings:** 2

- **Cooking Time:** 0 minutes

- **Nutritional Facts:** Approximately 100 calories per serving, high in vitamin C, hydration, and antioxidants.

- **Ingredients:**

  - 2 cups pineapple chunks

  - 1 cucumber, peeled

  - 1/4 cup fresh mint leaves

  - 1/2 lemon, peeled

- **Instructions:**

1. Pass pineapple chunks, cucumber, mint leaves, and lemon through a juicer.

2. Stir the juice well to combine.

3. Pour into glasses and serve immediately over ice if desired.

10. Carrot Ginger Orange Smoothie

- **Description:** Bright and zesty smoothie featuring carrots, oranges, and ginger for a refreshing and immune-boosting beverage.

- **Prep:** 5 minutes

- **Servings:** 2

- **Cooking Time:** 0 minutes

- **Nutritional Facts:** Approximately 150 calories per serving, high in vitamin C, beta-carotene, and antioxidants.

- **Ingredients:**

  - 2 large carrots, peeled and chopped

  - 2 oranges, peeled and segmented

  - 1/2-inch piece of ginger, peeled

  - 1/2 cup water or coconut water

- **Instructions:**

1. Place chopped carrots, orange segments, ginger, and water (or coconut water) in a blender.

2. Blend until smooth and creamy.

3. If the smoothie is too thick, add more liquid as needed and blend again until the desired consistency is reached.

4. Pour into glasses and serve immediately.

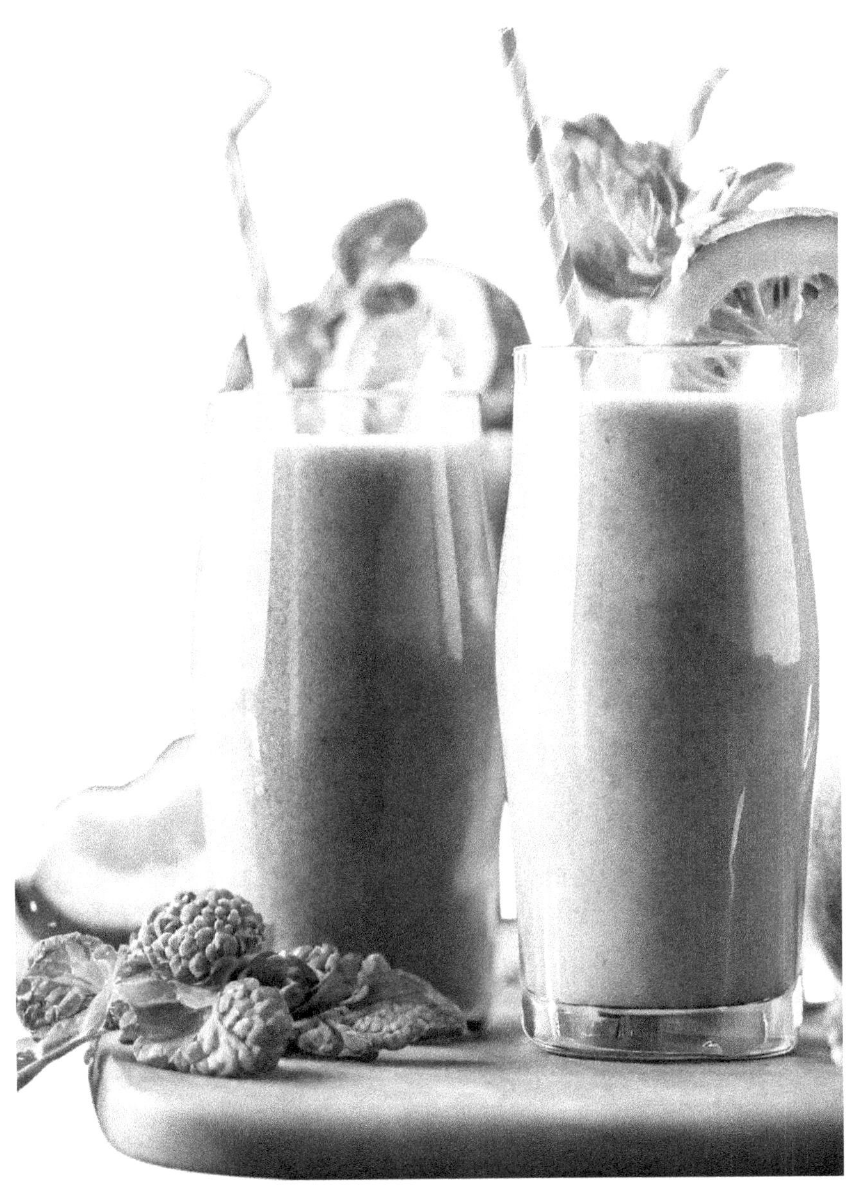

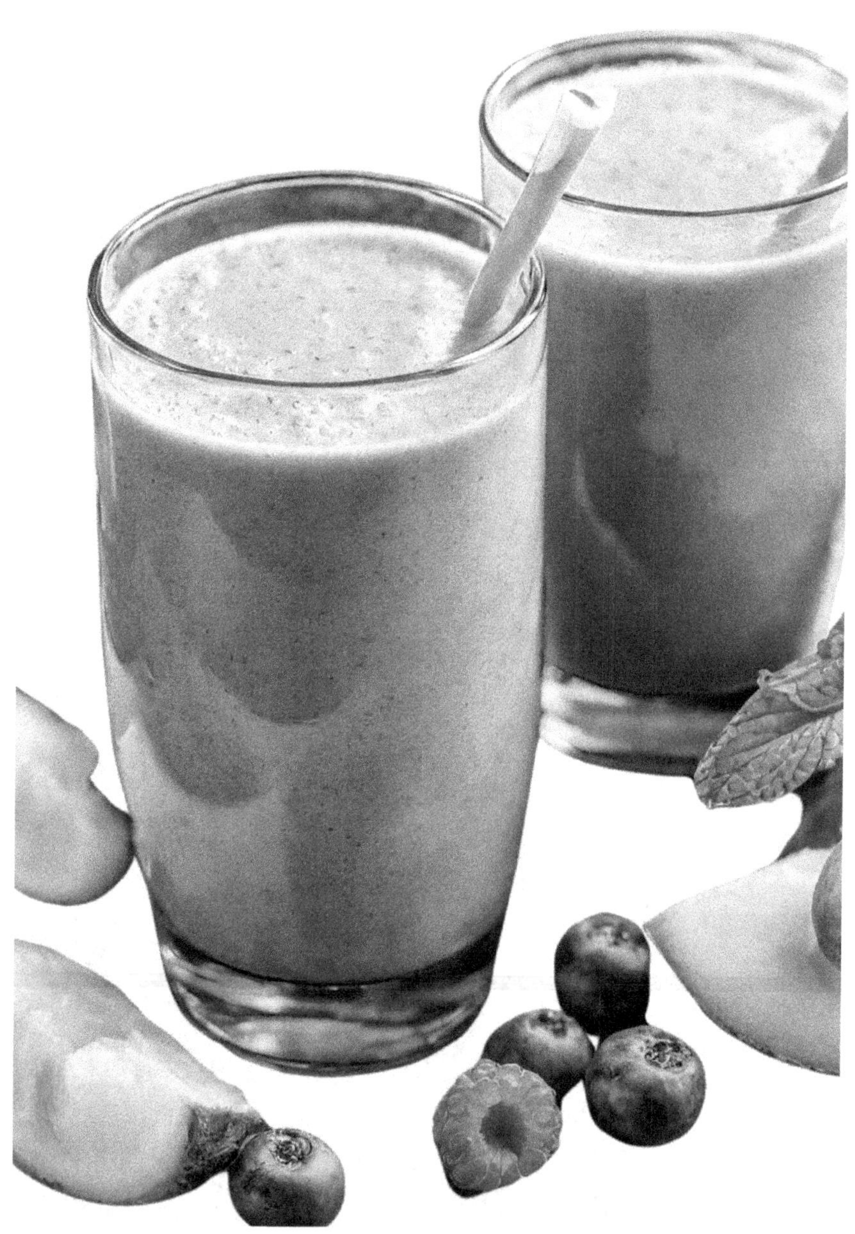

CHAPTER EIGHT

28-Day Meal Plan

Day 1:

Breakfast: Avocado Toast with Poached Egg

Lunch: Quinoa Salad with Chickpeas and Roasted Vegetables

Dinner: Baked Salmon with Steamed Broccoli and Brown Rice

Day 2:

Breakfast: Berry Spinach Smoothie

Lunch: Mediterranean Chickpea Salad

Dinner: Stir-fried tofu with Mixed Vegetables and Quinoa

Day 3:

Breakfast: Greek Yogurt Parfait with Granola and Berries

Lunch: Lentil Soup with Whole Grain Bread

Dinner: Grilled Chicken Breast with Roasted Sweet Potatoes and Asparagus

Day 4:

Breakfast: Veggie Omelet with Whole whole-grain toast
Lunch: Quinoa and Black Bean Stuffed Bell Peppers
Dinner: Shrimp Stir-Fry with Brown Rice

Day 5:

Breakfast: Overnight Oats with Almond Butter and Banana
Lunch: Chickpea Salad with Avocado Dressing
Dinner: Vegetable Stir-Fry with Tofu and Brown Rice

Day 6:

Breakfast: Whole Grain Pancakes with Mixed Berries
Lunch: Spinach and Strawberry Salad with Grilled Chicken
Dinner: Lentil and Vegetable Stir-Fry with Brown Rice

Day 7:

Breakfast: Breakfast Burrito with Scrambled Eggs and Avocado
Lunch: Greek Salad with Grilled Shrimp

Dinner: Turkey Meatballs with Marinara Sauce and Whole Wheat Pasta

Day 8:

Breakfast: Smoothie Bowl with Acai and Mixed Fruit
Lunch: Quinoa Salad with Roasted Vegetables and Feta
Dinner: Baked Chicken Thighs with Sweet Potato Mash and Steamed Green Beans

Day 9:

Breakfast: Mango Ginger Turmeric Smoothie
Lunch: Lentil and Kale Salad with Citrus Vinaigrette
Dinner: Baked Cod with Roasted Brussels Sprouts and Cauliflower

Day 10:

Breakfast: Banana Walnut Overnight Oats
Lunch: Greek Salad with Grilled Chicken
Dinner: Vegetable Stir-Fry with Tofu and Brown Rice

Day 11:

Breakfast: Blueberry Almond Smoothie

Lunch: Chickpea and Spinach Stuffed Bell Peppers

Dinner: Lentil and Vegetable Curry with Naan Bread

Day 12:

Breakfast: Peanut Butter Banana Smoothie Bowl

Lunch: Quinoa and Chickpea Salad with Lemon Tahini Dressing

Dinner: Turkey Meatballs with Marinara Sauce and Zucchini Noodles

Day 13:

Breakfast: Spinach and Mushroom Breakfast Burrito

Lunch: Lentil Soup with Whole Wheat Pita Bread

Dinner: Grilled Chicken Caesar Salad

Day 14:

Breakfast: Chia Seed Pudding with Mixed Berries

Lunch: Greek Salad with Grilled Shrimp

Dinner: Vegetable Stir-Fry with Tofu and Brown Rice

Day 15:

Breakfast: Avocado Toast with Poached Egg and Tomato Slices

Lunch: Quinoa and Black Bean Wrap with Greek Yogurt Dip

Dinner: Grilled Salmon with Mango Salsa and Wild Rice

Day 16:

Breakfast: Greek Yogurt Parfait with Granola and Mixed Berries

Lunch: Mediterranean Quinoa Salad with Grilled Chicken

Dinner: Baked Cod with Lemon Herb Butter and Roasted Vegetables

Day 17:

Breakfast: Banana Walnut Smoothie with Oatmeal

Lunch: Chickpea and Spinach Stuffed Bell Peppers

Dinner: Vegetable Stir-Fry with Tofu and Brown Rice Noodles

Day 18:

Breakfast: Blueberry Almond Overnight Oats

Lunch: Greek Salad with Grilled Chicken

Dinner: Lentil and Vegetable Curry with Naan Bread

Day 19:

Breakfast: Peanut Butter Banana Smoothie Bowl

Lunch: Quinoa and Chickpea Salad with Lemon Tahini Dressing

Dinner: Turkey Meatballs with Marinara Sauce and Zucchini Noodles

Day 20:

Breakfast: Spinach and Mushroom Breakfast Burrito

Lunch: Lentil Soup with Whole Wheat Pita Bread

Dinner: Grilled Chicken Caesar Salad

Day 21:

Breakfast: Chia Seed Pudding with Mixed Berries

Lunch: Greek Salad with Grilled Shrimp

Dinner: Vegetable Stir-Fry with Tofu and Brown Rice

Day 22:

Breakfast: Avocado Toast with Poached Egg and Tomato Slices

Lunch: Quinoa and Black Bean Wrap with Greek Yogurt Dip

Dinner: Baked Salmon with Mango Salsa and Wild Rice

Day 23:

Breakfast: Greek Yogurt Parfait with Granola and Mixed Berries

Lunch: Mediterranean Quinoa Salad with Grilled Chicken

Dinner: Baked Cod with Lemon Herb Butter and Roasted Vegetables

Day 24:

Breakfast: Banana Walnut Smoothie with Oatmeal

Lunch: Chickpea and Spinach Stuffed Bell Peppers

Dinner: Vegetable Stir-Fry with Tofu and Brown Rice Noodles

Day 25:

Breakfast: Blueberry Almond Overnight Oats

Lunch: Greek Salad with Grilled Chicken

Dinner: Lentil and Vegetable Curry with Naan Bread

Day 26:

Breakfast: Peanut Butter Banana Smoothie Bowl

Lunch: Quinoa and Chickpea Salad with Lemon Tahini Dressing

Dinner: Turkey Meatballs with Marinara Sauce and Zucchini Noodles

Day 27:

Breakfast: Spinach and Mushroom Breakfast Burrito

Lunch: Lentil Soup with Whole Wheat Pita Bread

Dinner: Grilled Chicken Caesar Salad

Day 28:

Breakfast: Chia Seed Pudding with Mixed Berries

Lunch: Greek Salad with Grilled Shrimp

Dinner: Vegetable Stir-Fry with Tofu and Brown Rice

CHAPTER NINE

The Value of Exercise in Cancer Prevention and Recovery

Regular exercise is important for both cancer prevention and rehabilitation. Here's why.

Reduces Cancer chance: Regular physical exercise may help lower the chance of getting some cancers, such as breast, colon, and lung cancer. Exercise promotes a healthy weight, which is associated with a decreased risk of cancer.

Improves Immune Function: Exercise strengthens the immune system, making it more capable of detecting and eliminating cancer cells. Regular physical exercise may also help decrease inflammation in the body, which has been related to the development of cancer.

Exercise may help decrease adverse symptoms associated with cancer treatment, such as tiredness, nausea, and depression. It may also enhance the overall quality of life throughout therapy.

Exercise improves recovery after cancer therapy by increasing strength, endurance, and mobility. It may also lower the chance of cancer recurrence and increase long-term survival rates.

To enjoy the advantages of exercise for cancer prevention and recovery, it's advised that you do at least 150 minutes of moderate-intensity aerobic activity or 75 minutes of vigorous-intensity aerobic activity each week, as well as muscle-strengthening exercises on two or more days each week.

Stress Management Strategies for Overall Wellness:

Stress management is critical for general health, particularly for those dealing with cancer or recovering from it. Here are some stress management strategies to consider:

Mindfulness meditation may help you decrease stress and relax. Concentrate on your breathing and examine your thoughts and feelings without judgment.

Deep Breathing Exercises: Incorporate deep breathing exercises into your everyday routine to trigger your body's relaxation response. Take slow, deep breaths, concentrating on filling your lungs with air before gently expelling.

Yoga and Tai Chi are moderate forms of exercise that incorporate physical movement, breath awareness, and meditation. These techniques may assist in relieving stress and promote general well-being.

Creative Expression: Use art, music, or writing to express your feelings and deal with stress. Creative hobbies may bring a feeling of satisfaction and relaxation.

Social Support: Seek out friends, relatives, or support groups to express your thoughts and emotions. Connecting with others who understand what you're going through may be calming and encouraging.

Healthy Lifestyle Habits: Put self-care first by leading a healthy lifestyle that includes frequent exercise, nutritious food, appropriate sleep, and limiting alcohol and caffeine use.

Putting these stress management tactics into your daily routine can help you deal with the difficulties of cancer diagnosis and treatment, as well as enhance your general quality of life.

Creating A Supportive Community for Your Health Journey:

Building a supportive environment is critical for coping with the hardships of cancer diagnosis and treatment. Here's why it matters:

A supportive community may give emotional support during tough times by empathizing, encouraging, and understanding. Connecting with individuals who have similar experiences might help to alleviate feelings of isolation and loneliness.

Practical aid: Friends, family, and support groups may provide practical aid such as transportation to appointments, assistance with domestic responsibilities, or food preparation during treatment.

Information and Resources: Being a member of a supportive community may offer you useful information and resources about cancer diagnosis, treatment choices, and local support services.

Empowerment and Advocacy: A supportive community can help you become an advocate for your own healthcare and treatment options. Sharing experiences and information allows you to become more educated and actively engage in your health journey.

To create a supportive network, try joining cancer support groups, engaging in online forums or social media groups, seeking assistance from friends and family, and connecting with local cancer organizations or services. Remember that you are not alone, and there are individuals ready to help you every step of the road. The Value of

Exercise in Cancer Prevention and Recovery:

Regular exercise is important for both cancer prevention and rehabilitation. Here's why.

Reduces Cancer chance: Regular physical exercise may help lower the chance of getting some cancers, such as breast, colon, and lung cancer. Exercise promotes a healthy weight, which is associated with a decreased risk of cancer.

Improves Immune Function: Exercise strengthens the immune system, making it more capable of detecting and eliminating cancer cells. Regular physical exercise may also help decrease inflammation in the body, which has been related to the development of cancer.

Exercise may help decrease adverse symptoms associated with cancer treatment, such as tiredness, nausea, and depression. It may also enhance the overall quality of life throughout therapy.

Exercise improves recovery after cancer therapy by increasing strength, endurance, and mobility. It may also lower the chance of cancer recurrence and increase long-term survival rates.

To enjoy the advantages of exercise for cancer prevention and recovery, it's advised that you do at least 150 minutes of moderate-intensity aerobic activity or 75 minutes of vigorous-intensity aerobic activity each week, as well as muscle-strengthening exercises on two or more days each week.

Stress Management Strategies for Overall Wellness

Stress management is critical for general health, particularly for those dealing with cancer or recovering from it. Here are some stress management strategies to consider:

Mindfulness meditation may help you decrease stress and relax. Concentrate on your breathing and examine your thoughts and feelings without judgment.

Deep Breathing Exercises: Incorporate deep breathing exercises into your everyday routine to trigger your body's relaxation response. Take slow, deep breaths, concentrating on filling your lungs with air before gently expelling.

Yoga and Tai Chi are moderate forms of exercise that incorporate physical movement, breath awareness, and meditation. These techniques may assist in relieving stress and promote general well-being.

Creative Expression: Use art, music, or writing to express your feelings and deal with stress. Creative hobbies may bring a feeling of satisfaction and relaxation.

Social Support: Seek out friends, relatives, or support groups to express your thoughts and emotions. Connecting with others who understand what you're going through may be calming and encouraging.

Healthy Lifestyle Habits: Put self-care first by leading a healthy lifestyle that includes frequent exercise, nutritious food, appropriate sleep, and limiting alcohol and caffeine use.

Putting these stress management tactics into your daily routine can help you deal with the difficulties of cancer diagnosis and treatment, as well as enhance your general quality of life.

Creating A Supportive Community for Your Health Journey

Building a supportive environment is critical for coping with the hardships of cancer diagnosis and treatment. Here's why it matters:

A supportive community may give emotional support during tough times by empathizing, encouraging, and understanding. Connecting with individuals who have similar experiences might help to alleviate feelings of isolation and loneliness.

Practical aid: Friends, family, and support groups may provide practical aid such as transportation to appointments, assistance with domestic responsibilities, or food preparation during treatment.

Information and Resources: Being a member of a supportive community may offer you useful information and resources about cancer diagnosis, treatment choices, and local support services.

Empowerment and Advocacy: A supportive community can help you become an advocate for your own healthcare and treatment options. Sharing experiences and information allows you to become more educated and actively engage in your health journey.

To create a supportive network, try joining cancer support groups, engaging in online forums or social media groups, seeking assistance from friends and family, and connecting with local cancer organizations or services.

In ending this Anti-cancer Diet Cookbook, we have gone on a journey together to discover the transforming potential of food in fighting cancer and strengthening our immune systems. We realized that the kitchen can be a refuge for healing and hope by creating comfortable and healthy foods that are specifically designed to assist our bodies.

As we say goodbye to these pages, let us carry on the information learned and the tastes enjoyed, knowing that each meal made with purpose has the power to nourish not only our bodies but also our souls. With each healthful ingredient and thoughtful culinary approach, we embrace the promise of a better future, full of vigor and resilience.

May this cookbook be a source of hope for everyone who wants to empower themselves in the battle against cancer, reminding us that the simple act of cooking has the deep capacity to alter our health and well-being? Let us continue to celebrate nature's richness and the healing power of tasty, nutrient-dense meals as we go forward with renewed drive and confidence. Together, we can fuel our bodies, fortify our immune systems, and eventually flourish in the face of hardship.

Good Luck In The Kitchen!

WEEK 1

MON

BREAKFAST	LUNCH	DINNER

TUES

BREAKFAST	LUNCH	DINNER

WED

BREAKFAST	LUNCH	DINNER

THURS

BREAKFAST	LUNCH	DINNER

FRI

BREAKFAST	LUNCH	DINNER

SAT

BREAKFAST	LUNCH	DINNER

SUN

BREAKFAST	LUNCH	DINNER

WEEK 2

	BREAKFAST	LUNCH	DINNER
MON			
TUES			
WED			
THURS			
FRI			
SAT			
SUN			

WEEK 3

	BREAKFAST	LUNCH	DINNER
MON			
TUES			
WED			
THURS			
FRI			
SAT			
SUN			

WEEK 4

	BREAKFAST	LUNCH	DINNER
MON			
TUES			
WED			
THURS			
FRI			
SAT			
SUN